Praise for *Scripts and Strategies in Hypnotherapy with Children*

Created from a combination of years of dedicated training and personal experience in practice, this book demonstrates the author's excellent understanding of the uniqueness and complexity of each young client and offers the reader a perfectly constructed springboard from which to execute their own individual therapeutic delivery.

The text is liberally salted with beautifully crafted example scripts that evoke the memories and imaginings of childhood so vividly that they may even address those unresolved issues that lurk within each of us as adult readers.

This is a totally accessible manual, written with an obvious passion and sensitivity for the needs of the child and mercifully avoiding the unnecessary use of technical language wherever possible.

The author states in her preface that "whether you already work with children or are just thinking of doing so, this book is aimed at you", and I can categorically confirm that she hits her mark with unnerving accuracy. I would also suggest that many therapists (and, by extension, their adult clients) are likely to benefit from this book even if they do not routinely work with children and consequently it would make a perfect addition to any practitioner's library.

William Broom, Chief Executive, The General Hypnotherapy Standards Council

At last, the book our profession has been waiting for, one those of us who know Lynda Hudson have been encouraging her to write for a long time. Lynda is the acknowledged expert on the use of hypnotherapy with children and her many years of experience are shared and reflected in the information, protocols, and creative and inventive scripts contained within this volume. Although aimed at the hypnotherapist, the broad spectrum of Lynda's work found herein will be of immense value to therapists of all disciplines, providing ideas, encouragement and that often sought after source of sensible advice. Although it may seem a cliché to say, *Scripts and Strategies in Hypnotherapy with Children* really is an essential addition to any therapist's library.

Peter Mabbutt, FBSCH, Director of Studies for the London College of Clinical Hypnosis, Co-author of *Hypnotherapy for Dummies*

This is a thorough, creatively composed and eminently practical book. Ms. Hudson has taken the principles of solution-focused therapy, oriented them skillfully towards the problems of children and adolescents and thereby produced myriad scripts and strategies that both illustrate and instruct. The scripts that form the heart of the book are appropriately nuanced and written flexibly allowing the clinician to adapt them to the individual child across a wide spectrum of clinical presentations. Hudson's enthusiastic, compassionate and affirming voice comes through the text of the scripts. I particularly appreciate the author's persistent emphasis on ego-strengthening and the modeling of permissive and responsive language which is central to hypnosis, particularly with young people. The framing of each set of scripts with an overview of the clinical problems for which they can be used, helpful strategies for engaging the child and parents, as well as extracts of the salient points of each chapter provide a unique depth to this text. Practical points for the parents of children with separation anxiety, the list of dissociation strategies, ego-strengthening guidelines and a host of other useful tips add to the book's value as a desk-side reference. Taken as a whole, this rich volume captures the confident, positive, warm and imaginative spirit that embodies creative hypnosis with young people then distills it into an enjoyable and practical solution. I will use it a lot.

Laurence I. Sugarman, MD,
President, American Board of Medical Hypnosis, Fellow, American Academy
of Pediatrics & American Society of Clinical Hypnosis, Clinical Associate
Professor of Pediatrics, University of Rochester School of Medicine and
Dentistry, Co-Author/Editor – *Therapeutic Hypnosis with Children and*
Adolescents, **Producer –** *Hypnosis in Pediatric Practice: Imaginative Medicine*
in Action

As a teacher/trainer of hypnotherapy practice for 37 years, I have seen many books which address aspects of the work. There has always been a gap in the available literature concerning the use of hypnotherapy with children.

Now, hypnotherapist Lynda Hudson's new book, *Scripts and Strategies in Hypnotherapy with Children,* supplies the much-needed approaches and techniques for working with children. Written without academic or scientific jargon, the many scripts for a great variety of juvenile problems are precise and useful tools. With the increasing recognition and growing popularity of hypnotherapy, parents are realising that medicating their children to modify behaviour is often a mistake. Behaviour is subject to change and hypnotherapy can quickly pinpoint and reshape the form and nature of it. Children respond to hypnosis more easily than many adults and respond to suggestions of change with enthusiasm. This is a book for every hypnotherapist's library, especially those who work with children or would like to learn how to work with them.

Gil Boyne, Executive Director, American Council of Hypnotist Examiners
Fellow, National Council for Hypnotherapy

Scripts and Strategies in Hypnotherapy with Children is a valuable resource for clinicians working hypnotically with children. Ms. Hudson's stories are delightfully imaginative; her language is permissive and she includes ego-strengthening in every script to foster self-esteem and self-efficacy.

The book offers the reader scripts and strategies for a variety of common pediatric problems including anxiety, sleeping problems, habit disorders, enuresis and encopresis. Robots, fairies, treasure hunts and space ships contained in the metaphors will all entertain the child while the carefully crafted therapeutic message is embedded in the story thus cleverly bypassing any resistance to change.

The strategies and scripts offered by Ms. Hudson can be used to enhance a clinician's existing area of expertise. The scripts are developmentally appropriate for the suggested ages and may be used verbatim or adjusted and incorporated into the clinician's own personal style. When working with children, the skilled practitioner must be flexible and open to the child's own creativity and spontaneity. Nearly anyone can learn how to induce a trance and certainly with children it is very easy, but the skilled and talented clinician will use the trance state to access the child's inherent strengths and resources. The true magic of therapeutic change lies with the child. They possess the creative genius. The success of providing the child with the tools to discover the magic and resources within depends in large part on the therapeutic relationship, rapport and alliance between the clinician and the child. Ms Hudson's book gives the clinician warm, caring and developmentally appropriate strategies that help foster rapport and successful hypnotherapeutic interventions with children. Ms. Hudson has provided the hypnosis world with a wonderful resource for working with children.

Linda Thomson, PhD, MSN, CPNP,
Author of *Harry the Hypno-potamus, Volumes 1 and 2*

I have often looked for a book like this on working with children, and this is an excellent volume. Lynda's easy to read style helps make this both an easy as well as an informative read. All-in-all a well structured and easy to read book which will form a welcome addition to any hypnosis practitioner's reference library.

Ursula James, Visiting Teaching Fellow, Oxford University Medical School
Honorary Lecturer at St Georges Medical School & Barts and the London
School of Medicine and Dentistry, PhD researcher – London Metropolitan
University, Author of the *Clinical Hypnosis Textbook*, *You Can Be Amazing*
and *You Can Think Yourself Thin*

Lynda Hudson is clearly an expert in her field. Here she has provided the hypnotherapist with a much needed comprehensive and practical guide to working with children. This book is an invaluable resource for any therapist and I highly recommend her strategies which I have used with great success in my own practise. This book will now be required reading for all our students of hypnotherapy.

Christina Mills, Founder and Director,
The Isis School of Integrated Hypnotherapy

This comprehensive handbook for hypnotherapists and other professionals in the health care sector provides an extensive collection of sparkling crystal clear scripts and strategies with a problem- and age-appropriate approach for 5–15-year-old youngsters. Any difficulties children of this age group may encounter on their way to further development, whether of a physical, mental, educational, emotional, or behavioural nature is richly provided for by tailor-made solution focused approaches. Lynda Hudson, a very experienced and highly professional therapist and lecturer, stresses repeatedly the importance of 'going with the flow' of information provided by the young clients themselves, speaking *their* language, using *their* learning style and adapting metaphors to *their* experiences so that the intervention is totally relevant to the child and therefore more powerful.

This unique handbook will provide professionals with many new, creative insights and suggestions to help relieve the difficulties so many youngsters and their immediate environment are experiencing.

Eleanor May-Brenneker MA, SpLDAPC

Those who treat children regularly will find this book a valuable addition to their bookshelf. It contains a wealth of useful advice, guidance and information when dealing with children and teenagers. It is clear, well written and comes from the pen of a therapist with great experience and skill in treating young people.

John S. Hempstead, Chairman, British Society of Clinical Hypnosis

Lynda Hudson's handbook does an admirable job in seamlessly integrating solution-focused and hypnotherapeutic approaches in providing a genuinely useful, clinically relevant, developmentally informed, practical source for hypnotherapists of all levels of experience working with children and young people.

The book offers a comprehensive collection of clinically informed, age appropriate hypnotherapeutic inductions and scripts which are easy to follow, individualise and implement. In addition the book contains advice on safe clinical practice and how to engage parents in treatment and provides useful references and websites.

This book will be of considerable interest for all hypnotherapists working with children and young people.

Karmen Slaveska-Hollis, MD,
Consultant in Child and Adolescent Psychiatry (MRCPsych)

Scripts and Strategies in Hypnotherapy with Children is a "must-read" for anyone who does hypnotherapy with children. The book is well-written. There are chapters on just about every childhood difficulty a therapist will encounter in working with children. Each of these chapters begins with an excellent summary of the condition involved (like self-esteem or encopresis). The hypnosis scripts are a joy to read since they incorporate hypnotic language usage of the highest order. The concepts of solution-focused brief therapy illuminate the scripts, as does the use of indirect (and direct where called for) language. Hudson obviously knows children and how to communicate with them. She also knows how to interact with parents to be able to enlist their cooperation and assistance in working with their child. The book is replete with common sense and practical advice for the practitioner. This is the best book of this type I have come across, and I cannot praise it too much. Hudson does not promise "cures," but rather that the use of hypnosis will assist the child to be more relaxed, more comfortable with themselves, and more functional in his/her world. The scripts are imaginative and clearly designed to intrigue and interest and provide the child with ideas for his/her own progress and happiness. This book will be a resource to be consulted over and over again by all those who use hypnosis with children. Highly recommended.

Rubin Battino, Author of *Ericksonian Approaches, Metaphoria, Coping,* *Expectation* **and** *Guided Imagery*

Scripts and Strategies in Hypnotherapy with Children

For use with children and young people aged 5 to 15

Lynda Hudson

Crown House Publishing Limited
www.crownhouse.co.uk
www.crownhousepublishing.com

First published by
Crown House Publishing Ltd
Crown Buildings, Bancyfelin, Carmarthen, Wales, SA33 5ND, UK
www.crownhouse.co.uk

and

Crown House Publishing Company LLC
PO Box 2223, Williston, VT 05495
www.crownhousepublishing.com

Mind Maps™ are a registered trademark of the Buzan Organisation

British Library Cataloguing-in-Publication Data
A catalogue entry for this book is available
from the British Library.

Print ISBN 978-184590139-4
Mobi ISBN 978-184590400-5
ePUB ISBN 978-184590241-4

LCCN 2008936804

Printed and bound in the UK by
TJ International, Padstow, Cornwall

For
Jonathon,
Frances and Tim

Table of Contents

Table of Scripts ii

Acknowledgements v

Preface.. vii

Chapter One   A Solution-Focused Approach 1

Chapter Two   Inductions...15

Chapter Three   Ego Strengthening and Self-esteem...........................29

Chapter Four   Nocturnal Enuresis 45

Chapter Five   Encopresis 59

Chapter Six   Tics and Habits...77

Chapter Seven   Anxiety 95

Chapter Eight   Separation Anxiety 125

Chapter Nine   Obsessive Thoughts and Compulsive Actions 137

Chapter Ten   Sleeping Difficulties..157

Chapter Eleven   Being Bullied..173

Chapter Twelve   Behaviour Problems...191

Chapter Thirteen   Learning and Exams..205

References and Useful Resources 227

Index 237

Table of Scripts

All ages given are approximate

Inductions
Resting story (5–7 years)..18
Talk to teddy (5–6 years)..19
Swinging hammock (6–10 years)..19
Your mind shows your body how to get heavier (12 years upward)......20
Relax and catch the numbers (12 years upward).......................21
Land of sweets/candy (6–11 years) 22
Hop onto a passing cloud (6–12 years) 23
Finger or hand levitation (10 years upward).............................24
Find the right place (10 years upward) 25
Pretend the chair has turned into a spaceship (5–8 years)......................25
Look at the light switch (8 years upward).................................26
Comfortable cushions (any age)..26

Ego Strengthening and Self-esteem
You are very special (5–9 years)...33
Be good at being yourself (6–12 years).......................................34
Compliments (any age)..34
You are a good friend (7/8 years upward) 35
Ladder of confidence (8–12 years)...37
Wash off harmful messages from the walls of your inner mind
   (10 years upward)..38
STOP messages on your mind computer (12 years upward) 40

Nocturnal Enuresis
Stay dry all night long (5/6–9 years)...53
Wake up and get up when you need the toilet (9 years upward)............54
Calm and stretch your bladder (8 years upward) 56

Encopresis
Poo in the toilet (4–6 years)...68
Robot help station (4–6/7 years) 70
Change your toilet habits (8–12 years) 72
Right time and place jigsaw (8–12/14 years) 74
Mr Smelly Poo (5/6–8 years) 76

Tics and Habits
Spaceship master controls (5–8 years) 82
You are in charge of your muscles (6/7–12 years)....................83
Turn off the tic (any age)..85
Noises or twitches (10 years upward) 87
Tic Script Extracts: 89
   Various suggestions dealing with: the urge to blink/the urge to
   clear the throat/embarrassment or shame/explaining the problem
   to others/dealing with other people's negative responses to you
Stop sucking your thumb (4–7/8 years)......................................92

Anxiety
Rewind procedure (any age)...105
Throw anxious feelings into the bin (4–8 years) 111
Lucky dip (5–8 years) 113
Treasure hunt (8–12 years).. 114
Worry castles in the sand (8–12 years)..................................... 117
Virtual reality (10 years upward) 119
Summary of Hypno-desensitisation procedure 121

Separation Anxiety
A selection of useful suggestions (different ages)....................131
Keep your thoughts in the right place (6–12 years) 133

Obsessive Thoughts and Compulsive Actions
Diminish the power of the unwanted thought (8/9 years upward) 143
Future time capsule (8–12 years)...145
Thought-stopping on your computer mind (12 years upward)............147
Wait before you act (10 years upward)......................................149
Trichotillomania hand levitation (10 years upward)................154

Sleeping Difficulties
Deal with unwanted night-time thoughts (9 years upward)..................166
Whisper away night-time worries (5–8/9 years)......................167
Sounds don't bother you at all (8–12 years) 169
Suggestions for fear of the dark..170

Being Bullied
Shrink the bully (6 years upward) 178
Protective bubble (verbal taunting or abuse) (8–12 years).....................178
Museum of your mind (Building confidence, resilience and positive
   thinking) (10/12 years upward)..180
Defeat the bully (8 years upward)...184
Cyber bullying (12 years upward) 187

Behaviour Problems
Good boy, well done (5–9 years) 198
Calm and polite (9/10–14 years) 199
Calm and well behaved in class (8/9–12 years).........................200
Congratulations on progress (5/6–8 years) 202
Manage change and disappointment (9/10 years upward)....................203

Learning and Exams
Listening and getting started (8/10–14 years) 213
Concentrate and stay focused (10 years upward).....................215
Improve your studying/reading for information skills (homework)
  (12 years upward)...218
Spelling strategy (adaptable to any age).................................221

Learning and Exams
Magic bus (Be confident for class work and tests)
  (adaptable to age 6–9 years)..222
Overcome exam nerves for older children (12 years upward)..............224

Acknowledgements

First and foremost I would like to thank my husband, John(athon) for all his wonderful belief and support, ideas and suggestions, and his patient reading, re-reading and yet more re-reading of the manuscript.

My other thanks go to:

- Dr Adam Skinner, paediatric anaesthetist at Melbourne Children's Hospital for his invaluable help in checking my facts, and giving advice and input on the medical aspects of problems. He has been most generous with his time and expertise, particularly as I know how pressured he is. Any mistakes that might remain (I hope there aren't any) are mine and not his

- Very importantly, the enchanting children who have attended my clinic over the last fifteen years; without them, this book would not have been written

- Jack and Tom Hudson for their helpful and enthusiastic trialling and advice on the suitability of scripts

- Ben (and Carolyn) for allowing me to discuss his treatment for ADHD

- Juliette Howe for her suggestion of The Land of Sweets

- Eleanor May for her input on Dyslexia; Julian Russell; Mary McGlynn; Del Hunter Morrill for inspiring certain ideas (see the references section)

- All the students on my training courses who sparked off ideas

- The friends, family and colleagues who have read and commented on my scripts and ideas, in particular Frances, and also

Paula, Klodi and Chris; for helpful design comments, Linda, Tim, Cath, Barbara, Christine, Nina, Avril and Anne

- NLP trainers Michael Neill and Ian McDermott, clinical Hypnosis trainer, Michael Joseph in the early nineties, without whom none of this would have happened

- Ursula James for her book *You Can Be Amazing* which encouraged me to 'get on with it' and finish the book

- At Crown House, David, for giving me no constraints, Bev and Rosalie for their work on my behalf and Tom for the cover design.

Preface

Working with children has been interesting, surprising, challenging, fun, rewarding and, above all, it continues to be a fascinating journey of learning. Each child I see teaches me something new and challenges the last assumption I made. Whether you already work with children or are just thinking of doing so, this book is aimed at you. Although you could read it straight through, I suggest that you read Chapters 1 and 2 first and then dip into the balance of material as needed. The book could also be used by medical or health practitioners who want to make use of gentle hypnotic techniques in their work. Many of these ideas have been discussed in the training courses I have given on 'Working with Children', and I thank all of the students who inspired new ideas from the contributions they made.

In the first chapter I consider some general issues and assumptions when working with children and I propose a useful solution-focused approach to structure each session. Subsequent chapters deal with the problems I have most frequently been asked to help children deal with over the last few years. All chapters begin with some discussion of background information, things to look out for and possible pitfalls to avoid. This section is followed by a selection of scripts, all of which have been used successfully, adapted and improved, many over the course of more than 10 years. Although different age ranges are suggested for each script, readers are encouraged to adapt the scripts as they see fit to suit the individual child in front of them. I have tried to offer several different scripts for each specific problem, in part to appeal to various thinking styles (visual, auditory and kinaesthetic), ages and interests, and in part because, in the real world, one script delivered on one visit is unlikely to be the final answer to any problem. This collection contains enough scope for two or three visits. I hope you will enjoy using, modifying and elaborating on these ideas as much as I have enjoyed developing them with my child patients over the years.

Within the scripts, **comments for the therapist** are in bold and set off by the symbol ☺ before and after the comment.

Pauses in the script are indicated by the ellipsis symbol ... .

Italics are used to show where to modulate your voice for additional emphasis in order to highlight embedded commands or particularly important phrases.

To my non British readers

As I am English and live in London, I have used largely British English vocabulary, spelling and expressions although I have offered some alternatives as I have gone along, e.g. 'candy' for 'sweets' and 'gotten' for 'got'. British spelling uses 'practice' for the noun and 'practise' for the verb so please don't think we have forgotten to proof read the text! I know in America you have 'Moms' and not 'Mums' and maybe you use 'good job' instead of 'well done' or 'brilliant'. It just becomes a little too unwieldy to try to include expressions to suit everybody but I hope you will feel free to adapt the text as you see fit for the particular child in front of you. Thank you for your understanding.

Lynda

Chapter One

A Solution-Focused Approach

Differences between Working with Children and Working with Adults

Children are usually very open to hypnotherapy and they generally have fewer misconceptions about it than do adults since children, the younger ones at least, have not seen or heard of stage hypnosis.

Perhaps the biggest differences in working with children are in the degree of formality employed in terms of the structure of the session, the techniques used and the style of interaction with the child. Children tend to be accustomed to using their imagination; they live in it on a daily basis, switching easily from being a dinosaur, to a knight, to a Dalek or to a nurse in a matter of minutes. When I ask children to see a picture of themselves at school, in their bedroom or at the dentist, for example, I rarely encounter the response I sometimes get from adults who say that they can't visualise the images or colours; children just do it. Similarly, if I ask a child to make a character bigger or smaller, it is done in a trice, which leads me to another difference in working with young people: the sessions often progress far more quickly than ones with adults.

Considerations

Always be prepared to use children's metaphors when they are offered, since theirs will generally be far more effective than any you have dreamed up in advance. Children will identify intensely with their own ideas, characters, language and metaphors and thus have a more personally meaningful experience when their ideas and vocabulary are accepted and used.

A child's age is an important factor to take into account, as it will affect his or her level of understanding of the concept of hypnosis. Having said this, chronological age can be very misleading; some 10 year olds are 'going on 16' and others are more like naive 8 year olds. Older children may have seen television programmes that show stage hypnosis, and so may have certain preconceptions about what is going to happen in the session. Think in advance about how you are going to explain to children what they are going to do and how the process will help them. Two or three stock ways of explaining the process to different age groups should be available. With younger children I usually talk in terms of having a 'special' part of their mind that is going to help them stop sucking their thumb or learn how to have dry beds while in a kind of daydream. Or I may ask them to play a special imagination game with me. If speaking to an older child, I generally use an explanation similar to the one I use with an adult perhaps substituting the words 'inner mind' for 'unconscious mind'. I find that almost everyone understands the concept of an unconscious mind when I interrupt what we are talking about to ask the name of their favourite TV programme or if they know their phone number. Once they have answered, I point out that, although they were not consciously thinking about it beforehand, the number was stored in their unconscious (or inner) mind along with other memories, feelings and the knowledge of how to do all kinds of things, such as walking, using the computer or sleeping. These examples can be changed according to the interests of child, his or her age and the presenting problem.

A child's ability or willingness to relax for long periods of time is, in part, determined by his or her age. Young children will wriggle about, often prefer to keep their eyes open, may physically act out your suggestions and appear far more 'awake' than their adult counterparts. They are likely happier engaging in a Neuro Linguistic Programming (NLP) procedure than in a standard 'adult' relaxing induction. At the same time, you can find exactly the opposite response. With the right degree of rapport, using the most appropriate induction for the individual child and given the right 'mood of the moment', even the youngest of children can surprise you by enjoying a deeply relaxed, even sleepy state of hypnosis. However, just because this has happened on one occasion, doesn't mean it will happen again the next visit. The same child may be less tired at the next session or just feel like having a more active interaction than before. The best advice is to always be on your toes and ready to swap a planned out approach for one that seems more appropriate at the time!

The age range I am focusing on in this book is from about 5 or 6 years old to 15 years old (although I have included the occasional script which could be used with children as young as 4 years old) but it is important to remember that anyone under the age of 18 years old is considered a minor in the eyes of the law in England and many other countries. I highly recommend that therapists working in private practice with children investigate and comply with the legal requirements and safeguards that apply in their own country. This step is essential for the protection of both the child and the therapist. For the safety and comfort of all concerned I am very happy to have a parent in the room, but I am careful to explain beforehand that generally I will be speaking to the child directly rather than about the child to the parent. This brings up another difference when treating children: parents and children may have different agendas regarding treatment goals and these may be either explicit or covert. For example, a child may feel perfectly happy just to improve classroom behaviour so as not to get into trouble at school whereas parents may feel that treatment has not been successful unless the child has stopped being difficult at home. It may be that such discrepancies need to be brought out into the open; how, when and where this is done will depend on individual circumstances.

When I speak to the parent initially, usually on the telephone, I explain that however young the child may be, it is important to set up the appointment so that the child *wants* to come. When children feel they are being dragged along against their will, they are unlikely to respond positively. I normally suggest that the parents say something along the lines of, 'We've spoken to somebody who has helped lots of other children to stop sucking their thumbs (or whatever the presenting problem may be) and she thinks she could help you too, but only if you want her to help you. What do you think?' This puts the onus of choice and responsibility on the child and lets the child know that you (the therapist) are on his or her side. In fact, when I first meet children I also check out that they really want me to help them, and it isn't just their parents who think it's a good idea. Normally, children are a bit surprised that I am asking and the interaction helps establish rapport.

Although it is important to sound confident about the likely success of treatment, words should be chosen carefully when talking to the child so as not to engender feelings of failure if the treatment doesn't work as quickly as expected, or indeed occasionally, does not have an effect at all. It is good to be confident but also include various possibilities: 'Usually children come to see me two or three times to sort out this kind of problem but everybody is different and you will do it in your own time and in your own way. Who knows, you might only need this one visit!'

It is important to explain the approach to parents before treatment begins and to gain their commitment to supporting the work to be done. This may mean practical support in terms of limiting drinks at bedtime in the case of nocturnal enuresis or it may mean more nuanced support in asking them to change the way they talk about the problem. A change of tense can be very significant; it can set the original problem firmly into the past and allow the possibility of change once the treatment has begun by simply learning to say, 'He *used* to wet the bed nearly every night' rather than, 'He *always wets* the bed every night'. It is also wise to explain that, although change sometimes comes immediately, it can also happen gradually with the occasional setback if a child is tired or unwell. It is important that parents avoid making negative statements such as, 'Oh, he's gone back to square one this week' and instead describe the situation in a way that doesn't defeat the child, such as, 'There have been a few blips this week because he hasn't been feeling well'. The most helpful thing parents can do is to acknowledge positive change wherever they notice it, and be supportive and not make an issue of it if there is little or no immediate change.

Summary: Things to do – Things to remember

To do:

- Check out legal and safety procedures and requirements when working with children.
- Prepare some age-appropriate explanations of hypnosis.
- Gain parental support for your approach between sessions.
- Speak directly *to the child* rather than *about the child* during the session.
- Use the child's own ideas.

Remember:

- Positive language is important.
- The session is more informal.
- Children show a willingness to use their imagination.
- The progress of the session can be extremely fast.
- Expect the unexpected.

A Word About the Solution-Focused Approach

The Brief Solution Focused Model of therapy was originated and developed in the 1980s by Steve de Shazer, Insoo Kim Berg, Larry Hopwood and Scott Miller at the Brief Family Therapy Center in Milwaukee, Wisconsin, in the United States. Steve de Shazer published the model in *Keys to Solution in Brief Therapy* (1985) and *Clues: Investigating Solutions in Brief Therapy* (1988). Here is not the place for a detailed discussion of the solution-focused approach but the interested reader will find a list of books and helpful websites at the end of the book. Suffice it to say that taking a generally forward-looking approach with children is very safe and will normally bring very positive results. In my opinion, general regression techniques are out of place with children except in special instances by those with very specific training and qualifications.

Basic Structure of a Solution-Focused Session within a Hypnotic Framework

When you use the following structure, adapting it, leaving out parts and doubling back as appropriate, you will find that the therapy is already taking place as you ask the questions. You will be putting across to clients that change is possible/likely/inevitable so that they fill in the details of the achievement scenario in their own minds. By the time you come to the hypnotic script, you may merely be reinforcing a change already made or, at least, begun.

Find Out About the Problem

- I spoke to your mum on the phone and she told me a bit about the problem as she sees it. Can you tell me a bit more about how you see it?

If the problem is embarrassing, such as bedwetting or soiling, it is better for you to mention it first in a matter-of-fact way so that it is easier for the child to talk about it. Ask parents beforehand how their young children refer to the problem and use their language where appropriate. Following are some examples of questions that appeal to different personalities, genders, ages or cultures.

- Your mum told me that although you don't have any problems in the daytime, you aren't having as many dry beds as you would like at night. Is that right?

- Mummy told me that sometimes your poos pop out into your pants without you noticing it. Does that happen more when you're busy playing or when you are watching TV? How would you like it if they only popped out when you want them to? How would it be if we try to find out more about when and where it happens so we can help you to feel more in charge?

Find Out What They Want To Achieve

As with adults, but perhaps particularly with children, it is important to wait to hear what a child has to say before making a hypothesis about cause and treatment. Listening actively will give you the required information and suggest a suitable strategy for the first treatment session.

- What would you like me to help you with today?

- In a perfect world what would you like me to help you do?

- If you had a magic wand, what would you want to happen?

- If you had three wishes to change the way things are, what would you wish for?

- Suppose we could ask the magic fairy to sprinkle fairy dust/ the wizard to cast his spell/Harry Potter to cast his spell, what would be different tomorrow?

- Suppose a miracle happens tonight when you're asleep and when you wake in the morning the problem is completely sorted out, what would be different?

- Suppose Father Christmas came early this year and sorted out this problem and that was his present to you, what would be different in your life?

- How will you know next week that it was worth coming to see me today? What will be happening that is different from before?

More Detailed Questions about the Achievement Scenario

- Once you have sorted out this problem, what will you notice first that is different? What then? What next? How does that make a difference to you? What's better about that now? How is that better for you? *(Notice the deliberate shift to the present tense, which has the effect of encouraging the mindset that change is possible.)*

- What else will have changed? (Translate absence of symptoms into beginnings of new behaviours, for example, 'Oh, so you won't be frightened of going into school now. That's good. How will you be feeling instead? Will this mean you can walk in on your own or will you be chatting with your friends? What will you be doing instead of crying?')

Relationship Questions that Further Enrich the Achievement Scenario and Allow You to See the Family's Attitude and Reactions

- What will your mum/dad/best friend/grandma/sister/ brother/teacher/teddy/dog/worst enemy see you doing that will let them know that you have made an amazing change?

7

Work through a good selection of these questions, making sure to include people the child has told you are important.

- What will you notice that's different about your mum/dad now that this change has happened/now that you are having more dry nights/now that you aren't sucking your thumb/ now that you aren't pushing your sister anymore?

- Who else will notice the change? What will they think/feel/ say?

Ask questions that include a mix of visual, auditory and kinaes-thetic modalities to ensure maximum appeal and involvement in all the senses.

Exception Questions

- Are there times when some of this already happens/the spell already works/small parts of the miracle already happen/ things go just the way you want them to/you already know how to do this?

Exception questions are very important as they provide informa-tion about when, where or why a problem-behaviour does or does not occur already. Answers here will allow you to discover useful strengths, qualities or behaviours that the child already possesses or uses. If the child doesn't provide answers, you can set a 'notic-ing task' for homework, for example, 'What I'd like you to do over the next week is just to notice all the times when you manage to control your temper and come back and tell me about them next week. Will you do that?' Not only are you giving the child a posi-tive 'noticing task', you are also offering an implicit suggestion that there will indeed be times when he or she manages to carry out the desired behaviour.

Scaling Questions

- On a scale of 0 to 10, where 10 means the nervous feelings are the worst they've ever been and zero is when you are com-pletely laid back and calm, where are you now? (*Or you can reverse the numbering system since children often prefer to move up a scale rather than down.)*

You can scale any kind of behaviour, thought or emotion and this gives you useful initial information. It can also mark the progress in the next session: 'Last week you were at 9, where are you now?' It can allow all kinds of other questions to be used that help move the patient forward such as, 'If you are at 5 now, and at 10 you wouldn't be nervous at all, what would be different if you were at 7?' This question breaks down the goal into smaller steps that may be more realistic and more manageable. You can use prediction questions such as, 'Brilliant! You've gone from 3 to 5 in a week! What number do you think you are going to be on next week when you come back to see me? Oh, great. You'll be at 6 and a half. What will you be doing differently when you are at 6 and a half?'

You can use scaling with much younger children too; you can draw a hill on a flipchart or page and give them the pen to show you how far up the hill they will be next time they see you. You can simply get them to show you with their hands how high or low they will be or have them build a tower of bricks. You can use your imagination to think of other examples but best of all, you can use theirs. They are likely to be even more imaginative than you are and the whole interaction becomes an enjoyable game in which they are already stretching or breaking through their comfort zones.

'Anything Else?' Question

Before moving on to any hypnotic intervention, it is useful to ask one of the questions below. It is sometimes the answer to this question that yields the most enlightening piece of the jigsaw puzzle, the one that helps you to conclude the therapy successfully.

- Is there anything else you wanted to tell me that I didn't ask?

- Is there anything else important that you think I should know/I forgot to ask you about?

- Sometimes the tiny things are the really, really important things. Are there any tiny things you can tell me that I didn't ask you about?

9

Hypnotic Intervention of Your Choice

Example of an intervention suitable for almost any treatment session

- Compliment the child on his or her part in the session.

- Gentle 'day-dreamy' induction (see Chapter 2). (Or you may choose to use a visualisation or NLP technique with no induction.)

- A means of letting go of worries and anxious feelings (see Chapter 7).

- Guided imagery of the achievement scenario using all the personal information you have gained in your solution-focused questioning.

- Find a way to include compliments on the child's strengths/ qualities that will be instrumental in achieving the goal.

Set a Suitable Homework Activity

- A 'Noticing' Task:
  - Notice what happens when you drink lots and lots of water during the day but don't drink after 7 o'clock.
  - Notice how your teacher reacts when you stop pushing your classmates.

- Spend 2 minutes before you go to sleep imagining exactly what you *want* to happen (*not* what you *don't* want to happen).

- Listen to a supporting CD every night (if you have made one or suggested one) (see Resource Section).

- Suggest that they do something different this week without telling anybody what they are doing. See how it alters the problem and see if anybody else notices. Offer an example of something carried out by another child in a different situation so they understand what you mean: 'Somebody I know decided to count to 10 before answering his dad back just to see what difference it made' or 'Somebody else decided to put her hand up instead of calling out in class just to see how long it took the teacher to notice'.

Why Give Homework Activities?

Giving homework activities can help in several different ways; it speeds up the rate of progress and it helps children understand that the responsibility for change also lies with them and not wholly with you. 'Noticing activities' can uncover previously unrecognised critical information as in the case of one little boy who discovered that whenever his mother put him to bed he wet the bed, but when his father did it he was nearly always dry. It came out that there were difficulties in the marriage and the child felt more secure when the father was a part of the bedtime routine. Sometimes the suggestion to 'notice what happens with your dad/ teacher/sister when you try something different' places the focus on the fun of noticing other people's responses to the new behaviour, thus bypassing resistance to the new behaviour itself.

Positive visualisation can bring about seemingly miraculous improvement and restricting it to 2 minutes at bedtime will usually ensure that it is carried out. Sometimes asking children to devise their own homework can encourage identification with the exercises and increase their commitment to engaging in the activity.

I find that giving the child a recording of the hypnotic part of the session can be invaluable if the intervention is suitable for repeated listening as is, for example, the case with guided visualisation of the desired behaviour and ego boosting. If you do not have recording facilities, consider providing or recommending a published CD. The ones I have recorded for children are available on my website.* The provision of a CD is a particularly good idea when the child in question would greatly benefit from relaxation and relief from tension but finds it difficult to relax in the session. Listening to the CD at bedtime when the child is beginning to wind down anyway can accustom him or her to the process of relaxing and developing a day-dreamy state. The state may then be easier to replicate in subsequent sessions with you.

---

* www.firstwayforward.com

Supportive Message

A very effective strategy to use with children who need quite a lot of support, or when there are going to be extended gaps between visits, is to send an email or letter outlining or reminding them of a homework activity or offering a supportive message. We all like to receive mail and children are particularly delighted with it. A card simply saying how brilliantly a child responded in the session can work wonders for rapport and willingness to engage fully in the treatment next time.

EARS procedure

Use this structure for the second appointment and any subsequent appointments.

Elicit

- 'What's better/different from before?'
- Go through the different days.

Amplify

- Flag changes verbally and non-verbally.
- Use questions to expand on how change occurred, e.g., 'Great! Did that surprise you/your mum/your sister?'
- 'So, how did you feel that morning?'
- 'What difference did that make to your day?'
- 'What else was different? How did that help you?'

Restate

- 'So, you woke up and *the dry bed* was the first thing you noticed?'
- 'So, you got up, *went to the bathroom* and suddenly realised that *your bed was dry*! How did you feel about that?/That must have felt great, didn't it?'

Start again

- 'What else has been different? How many other ways has this made your life different?'

Use your chosen hypnotic script or intervention. Always include some kind of ego strengthening and congratulations for progress, however little it may have been.

Chapter Two

Inductions

Considerations When Choosing or Writing Scripts for Young People

When choosing or writing a script it is important to bear in mind the age of the child with whom you are working. It is also important to remember that chronological age is not necessarily an indicator of emotional maturity. If you choose something that is too young for an adolescent, for example, you not only risk losing the young client's interest, you risk alienating him or her altogether. Interestingly, these older clients will often respond enthusiastically to ideas that you originally conceived for younger children once you have won them over, but on a first occasion it is really crucial to try to strike the right note. For the 12 to 15-year-old age bracket, it is better to err on the side of overestimating rather than underestimating the client's maturity if there is any doubt.

The comments from Jack, nearly 10 years old and Tom, 7 years old, illustrate how important it is to 'get it right' for the age group. I was trialling one of my pre-publication CDs with them: Tom described it as 'Stupid and boring!' whereas his brother, Jack, responded with, 'Brilliant. Spot on!' More trialling confirmed that the suitable age group for the particular CD was 10–14!

In the writing of this book, every time I find myself thinking of making some general statement, an example instantly springs to mind that contradicts what I was about to say. This in itself underscores the fact that when you work with children you need to be constantly on your toes and prepared to move from one approach to another even in mid-flow! Still, generally speaking I would say that the younger children are, the shorter the script should be (10 to 15 minutes maximum). The best approach with really young ones is just to tell them a metaphorical story with embedded suggestions for the desired outcome. You can simply begin with suggestions for settling down and getting comfy. The more interactive the story, the better:

'Imagine you are just going to go into a magic garden. Does it have a gate? (Yes) What colour is it? (Blue) Are there flowers in your garden, Katie? (Big red ones) I see, so you've just pushed open the little blue gate and you can see the big red flowers in front of you … Are they the biggest, brightest, reddest flowers you've ever seen? Fantastic! Now, notice how springy the grass is under your feet.'

Whatever the age, just using the child's name has a very powerful effect, particularly if you have recorded the session or the script to listen to again at home. Children often tell me how much they enjoy hearing their name used.

I have found that the older children are the more patience they have with the idea of a typical relaxing induction; on the other hand, the younger the children the more you need to engage their imagination right away. There is no need to be concerned when young children move around and keep their eyes open: the goal is to get them imaginatively involved rather than to have them deeply relaxed. Having said that, there have been occasions when I have had very young children of 4 or 5 years old relax so deeply that they have drifted off to sleep. Incidentally, if that should happen, always ask a parent to be the one to rouse the child so that he or she is not completely disoriented upon waking.

Over the years I have noticed that girls and boys tend to have different preferences and different responses to approaches. I find that boys may wriggle about more than girls, and they tend to be more interested in the practical and technical side of things. Of course, some girls love to imagine themselves on a football field and some boys love the feeling of snuggling up all comfy and cosy on the settee, so the best advice is to listen carefully to their answers to your questions. In other words, always respond very directly to the child in front of you.

Summary

Age affects:

- understanding of concepts.
- understanding of specific vocabulary.
- ability to listen for a long time.
- interest.
- ability to relax.
- need to wriggle about.
- willingness to close eyes.

Gender *may* affect:

- physical presentation.
- the prevalence of presenting problems.
- interest in different topics.

Inductions for Different Age Groups

Nearly all of the following inductions can be used equally well as deepeners, but remember that mental engagement rather than depth of trance is the objective with younger children. The use of more than one induction or deepener might be too challenging/ testing for very young, short attention spans and so be counter-productive. The best advice is to be prepared for some trial and error, accompanied by acute observation and flexibility, and even then to remember how much children vary in individual likes and dislikes.

You can see examples elsewhere in the book of how some of the following inductions can be used to lead into complete scripts dealing with specific problems. All ages given are approximate and scripts can and should be adapted as necessary.

To avoid misunderstanding by child or parent I suggest using verbal rather than tactile inductions unless you are a medical practitioner or a therapist who uses touch as part of your main therapy, such as in physiotherapy. This is not to say that tactile inductions do not work well because they can be amazingly good ways to induce trance, but they can also be open to misinterpreta-tion. If you do use them, be certain to explain in advance to both parents and children that you may lift their hand or arm, or touch their forehead. These gestures should only be done with a parent present in the room. Given this caution, I have included only one script that has reference to lifting a child's arm and letting it drop.

Induction Script: Resting story

Age range: approximately 5–7 years

This is your very own resting story … I wonder if you know how to rest, really rest I mean? … I wonder if you could pretend that *you are really resting* so well that if someone were to look at you they would think *you are nearly asleep* … I wonder if *your arms are all floppy* … and if your legs are all floppy …

⌒ **Continue with hands, feet, eyelids, etc., using as many or as few suggestions as needed.** ⌒

It's good to feel drowsy/sleepy and comfy as you snuggle down while you daydream … or even night dream … because we all like to *dream and feel safe* and *feel comfy and even a bit sleepy* … and I wonder where you *first begin to feel that gentle warm, comfortable sleepy feeling* spreading around your body … does it *start at the top of your head and go all the way down your body*, down to the very tips of your toes? … or, is it the other way around, do your feet get warmer first and then let the comfy feelings spread all the way up to the top of your head? … Or does it seem to *spread out from the middle of your tummy?* … so you *feel comfy on the inside, comfy on the outside, inside out* … and comfy all over all the way through, that's right, that's wonderful … So I think now you are really ready to hear your resting story.

Variation on a theme: Pretend to be asleep

Relaxing is a bit like pretending to be asleep. Can you pretend? … Let's see if you can pretend so well that you really look as if *you are asleep right now* … Pretend that *you are so sleepy* your *whole arm has become really heavy and floppy* … Pretend that *your arm is so heavy* that if I pick it up and let it go … *it will just flop down completely* just as if *you are fast asleep right now.*

⌒ **Continue with legs, hands, etc., as necessary. You can omit the lifting and dropping of the arm if you prefer.** ⌒

Induction Script: Talk to teddy

Age range: approximately 5–6 years

Use any toy/doll/teddy and talk to them instead of the child, including embedded suggestions as you talk.

> I'm so glad (Child's Name) that you brought teddy along with you today because teddies are usually brilliant at relaxing … shall we see how well *your* teddy *can relax right now*? … So … teddy, can you *let one of your arms go really floppy now* … just as if *your arm is asleep* … that's amazing teddy … *really heavy and floppy* … and how about your other arm? Can you *let that one go all floppy too*? … almost as if *your arms are too heavy and sleepy to move* … hey, you're wonderful at doing this … and what about your legs … I bet your legs will *feel even heavier* than your arms when you *let them go all floppy and tired too* … and teddy do you think that (Child's Name) can let his/her body go floppier than yours and *be really, really still* or do you think that *you are the best* … *you are so floppy* that if anybody looked at you they would think *you are fast, fast asleep* … brilliant … *you are both fantastic at this.*

Variation on a theme: Ask the child to teach teddy how to relax

> I think (Child's Name) that you could show teddy how to relax today because mummy tells me that you are brilliant at relaxing when you go to bed … shall we see how well your teddy *can relax right now*? … Will you show him how to do it a little bit at a time? … Show him how to let one of his arms go really floppy … that's it … is his arm as floppy as yours? … Great … now show him how to relax his other arm and see if he can be nearly as good as you.

> ✆ Continue in this way until you get the degree of relaxation that you are looking for. ✆

Induction Script: Swinging hammock

Age range: approximately 6–10 years

> ✆ Make sure that the child understands the meaning of the word 'hammock' or show a picture first. ✆

> Make yourself (Child's Name) nice and comfy in the chair because you'll want to *feel very comfortable* while you listen and let your mind *drift off to the place where you like to daydream* and, later night dream … a nice, happy place where you can *feel very, very comfortable* … comfortable in yourself, comfortable about yourself in every way.

> Is that place somewhere you know? … Somewhere you've been or just somewhere happy and calm inside you? … And it's good to *feel (drowsy and) comfy as you settle down…* while you daydream … because we all like to *dream and*

19

feel safe … and feel comfy and even a bit sleepy … and I wonder where you *first begin to feel that gentle warm, comfortable sleepy feeling* spreading around your body? … Is it in your feet and your toes? … Or is it in your hands and your fingers? … Is it in your lower legs or your upper legs? … Wherever it is, you can just *enjoy feeling so comfy now* … feeling even comfy enough to imagine that you are in a hammock … imagining your body swinging gently backwards and forwards, just melting into relaxation … backwards and forwards … that's right … (Child's Name) melting into relaxation.

And you know what a hammock is like … it's made of rope and very strong net so that as you swing, you know *you are very, very safe* … your body swinging gently backwards and forwards, just melting into relaxation … backwards and forwards … that's right … and as you swing, any *old tight unwanted feelings just drift away* and out through the holes in the netting of the hammock … *your body is getting more and more comfy*, more and more relaxed and calm … any old worries … you can just breathe them away … and they too just disappear through the holes in the hammock … so you can *feel completely calm and comfortable* … that's right, just breathe them away now.

Induction Script: Your mind shows your body how to get heavier

Age range: approximately 12 years upward

This is a useful kinaesthetic introduction to any script that includes the idea of the mind taking unconscious control of the body, as in cases when the goal is to stop nail biting or thumb sucking, for example.

Make yourself comfortable and allow your eyes to close … and as you sit there, (Child's Name) just listening to the sound of my voice … and letting all the muscles of your body relax … becoming really aware of just how powerful your mind really is … I'm wondering if you know you can *use your mind to show your body what to do?* … Just say to yourself mentally and silently, *really* meaning it, *my left arm is getting heavier and heavier* … and then notice how your arm follows your thought and begins to *feel heavier and heavier all on its own* … *that's right* … now try it with your right arm, say to yourself … *my right arm is getting heavier and heavier...* and then *notice how that arm is getting heavier and heavier … more and more comfortable* … isn't that interesting how your own mind can direct your body? … Now try it with your left leg and find it *getting heavier and heavier too, getting heavier* and heavier … that's right … now try it with your right leg and find it too getting heavier and heavier, getting heavier and heavier … that's right, brilliant … and you can *continue doing this* with each word I speak and with each breath you take … becoming more and more relaxed … feeling more and more comfortable … feeling more and more relaxed … *even more comfortable* than before … that's right, that's brilliant.

And in this comfortable slightly dreamy state, I want to talk to you (Child's Name) about your mind ... which is so incredibly clever ... we all have a very special part of our mind and we call this part *your special* ... inner ... mind ... this is the part of the mind that controls all the things your body does automatically like breathing, for example ... without your ever having to tell it to do it for you ... even when you are fast asleep *you breathe easily and well* ... and this inside part of your mind is always looking after you ... wherever you are.

Induction Script: Relax and catch the numbers

Age range: approximately 12 years upward

And as you sit there and *listen to the sound of my voice* ... maybe you (Child's Name) can focus your eyes on that light switch over there ... instead of looking at me or getting distracted by the stuff in the room ... *you are in complete control* of whether you choose to stay looking at that light switch ... ☜ **If at this point the child chooses to keep eyes open, you have given him or her something on which to focus attention rather than having him or her look directly at you or being distracted by other things in the room.** ☜ or whether you *want to allow your eyes to close* whenever *they feel like closing* ... whenever they feel like it will be absolutely fine ... I want you to know there's no right way to do this ... and there's no wrong way ... whichever way you do *it, will be perfect for you.*

☜ **You are removing any possible worries about 'having to get it right'.** ☜

Some people just *like to increase* their *focus* ... and other people *like to relax* ... some people like to *relax a little* ... and some people like to *relax a lot* ... and some people like to *relax a little and then relax a lot...* whatever *you* do, will *be perfect for you* ... and as you *think about it* and *really notice now...* I wonder *which leg seems heavier* ... and *seems more relaxed than the other one?* ... And as you *shift your attention now* ... I wonder *which arm seems heavier* ... and which arm *seems more relaxed than the other?* ... Or if it's just *too much effort to bother noticing* ... as you are becoming aware that this is the *time to release the calm inside* ... and *do know that you have that calm and confidence inside* ... *so* settling yourself down now ... calm and confidence drifting up to the surface.

And now you are going to hear me count from 10 to 1 ... each number will help you to increase your ability to focus ... and become really ready to *take on board all the positive suggestions* that are right for you so you will be able to feel confident/feel calm and at ease/drift off to sleep just as you told me you want to.

So ready now, as I count ... maybe you will see the numbers in your mind's eye change ... and maybe you will see if you can catch the numbers before they change ... 10 ... See it change to 9, calm and comfortable ... 8, that's right ... I'm wondering whether you are catching the numbers or whether they're slipping through your fingers as they change ... more and more calm and comfortable ... changing to 7 ... and as you notice the comfort and as you notice the calm, you notice it spreading with each outward breath ... 6, and as the calm increases so you become aware of a clear and alert focus developing ... 5, you can see things very clearly ... 4 ... 3 ... 2, you are clear, alert and focused ... 1, that's right.

Now, in this ideal state, your mind has been becoming very, very attentive and eager to receive all the positive suggestions that you and I agreed would be good for you ... and are what you really want.

Induction Script: Land of sweets/candy

Age range: approximately 6–11 years

This introduction was inspired by an 11-year-old girl named Juliet, who described to me where she went in her mind as she daydreamed before she went to sleep. Bear in mind that this would not be a suitable induction for a child who is either overweight or whose parents don't allow him or her to eat sweets.

Make yourself comfortable and allow your eyelids to close ... you may *feel that this is the perfect time for a daydream* ... and the wonderful thing about a daydream is that *your imagination can take you anywhere wonderful you want to go* ... and as you *daydream here of lying in your bed* ... drifting and day-dreaming ... you can remember that your bedroom leads to a very special land ... the land of sweets/candy ... there's a very special (trap) door ... and when you *open it* ... you will find that it leads to a slide/chute ... can you see it? ... How about just sitting on the top of it now? ... And before you slide down to the land of sweets ... as you sit on the top ... you can *wonder exactly where-abouts you are going to land today* ... will it be on the bank of marshmallows? ... All soft and squashy ... or will it be on the candy floss/cotton candy/fairy floss meadow? ... All fluffy and light ... or could it be into the milkshake pool? ... Every time you slide down you could land somewhere different, you know ... the only thing you know for sure is that you will have a very safe and sweet landing ... and if you should land in the milkshake pool ... well ... of course, all you have to do is to give yourself a good shake ... maybe that's why it's called a milk 'shake' pool ... and you will be completely dry ... so why not slide down right now ... that's right ... and when *you've landed somewhere wonderful* you can nod your head and let me know.

Ideas for development of the theme

Go to the smoothie/juicer bar where worries or bad habits are like fruit pips which are strained and not allowed through into the drink itself.

Mix all the appropriate ingredients to make positive popcorn/confident candy/ chilled out chews/calm caramels, which they can eat for the appropriate effect.

Take them to a gingerbread house where they could meet a wise person who gives them advice.

Break pieces off the gingerbread house and eat them. Each piece has a different function, e.g., the windows help you see things more clearly, foundations and walls help you feel strong, and chimneys help let angry feelings come out.

Induction Script: Hop onto a passing cloud

Age range: approximately 6–12 years

Always take care before selecting sky/cloud inductions that the child doesn't have any associations with dying and going to heaven, a place in the sky. If you feel the child would prefer it, you can add in safety belts and harnesses, but most children I have come across seem perfectly happy just to hold onto the balloon string and float!

> And as you relax so comfortably there, I wonder just how quickly your creative mind can drift off to a place where the sun is shining … there's some green, green grass … could be a field … could be a park or a riverbank perhaps … could even be a lovely garden … and as you look around you here … you can feel the warmth of the sun on your skin … you can hear a gentle breeze rustling through the leaves of the trees … and as you look up into the blue sky … can you notice a few fluffy white clouds drifting along? … And look … as well as the clouds … there are some brightly coloured balloons too … and hey … quite a lot of the balloons have got children holding onto the strings … they're being carried along by the gentle breeze … floating happily along … they're having a great time … look behind you … and you will see that there are more balloons floating past … you can grab a string if you want to … just like the other children … and the balloon will float you along up into the sky … you can go whichever way you want just by pulling on the string this way … or … pulling on it that way … try it out … that's right … you can go just as quickly as you want … zooming along … or … just as slowly as you want … you can stay as low or as high as you want … drifting … floating … not a care in the world … feeling light and happy … noticing clouds drifting past from time to time … all fluffy and white … a bit like white candy floss/cotton candy/fairy floss … there's one cloud with some children sitting on it … they're looking very happy … one of them is calling out to you …. 'Why don't you hop onto a cloud? … It can take you somewhere wonderful.' … So … hop onto a passing cloud … and see where it will take you … that's it … feel how comfortable that is … you can relax right back into it and it supports/holds you beautifully.

🦀 Take the child off to a suitable place to receive your posthypnotic suggestions. Worries, unwanted habits and feelings could be allowed to float
away as he or she goes. 🦀

Induction script: Finger or hand levitation

Age range: approximately 10 years upward

This script appeals to both visual and kinaesthetic senses.

This is a standard finger or hand levitation script to be found in many, many
books and training courses but I have included it here because it is so simple
and easy to use and yet so powerful, especially with teenagers. I will often use it
as a very quick induction into a second 2-or-3-minute trance state, after having
brought them out of the main trance. In this second trance I suggest that, since
the unconscious mind clearly has the power to lift the fingers or hand off the lap,
it certainly has the power to carry out all the desired suggestions they have just
heard.

🦀 **Ask the child to let his or her fingertips rest lightly on his or her lap,
barely touching, and to fix all attention on the fingers.** 🦀

As you *look at that hand* and *keep staring at that hand*, I'd like you to begin to
really notice it in a way you've never done before … see just what *is different*
from before … is it becoming a bit fuzzy and a bit blurred? … Is there a kind of
outline around the hand? … Or, around the fingers?

It doesn't actually matter what you see or what you don't see … as long as you
notice what you see or notice what you don't *see right now* … notice how you
feel the difference too … notice what you feel and notice what you don't feel …
and … *yes, that's it* … I'd like you to notice that something has probably been
changing in your fingers now as you listen.

Can you *notice that your fingers* … right at the tips of your fingers … *are feeling a kind of tingling feeling* … *feeling lighter and lighter* … wanting to *lift off
your lap?* … Yes, that's great, that's amazing that your inner mind/special part
of your brain is so powerful … is so strong that it can *lift your fingers right off
your lap* all on their own … without your doing anything to help them at all …
they're lifting all on their own … hey, you're amazing.

And as your fingers get lighter so you may have noticed that your eyelids have
been getting heavier too. 🦀 **Continue in this vein until you have achieved
the desired effect.** 🦀

Induction Script: Find the right place

Age range: approximately 10 years upward

This may be the right time for you to take a few minutes to relax and do some-thing just for you … nobody else but you … feel good about you … here in this place … and there usually *is a right time and a right place for everybody … a right place for everything* … a space where you can *think differently* … a time where you can *see things in a new way* … where you can *feel more calm and at ease* … and *things seem to fall into place* … all on their own.

So let's see if we can *find that place … find exactly the right place … for you* … where you know what you really want in your life … and what you don't want … maybe it's a place you know … a place you've been … or maybe it's just a wonderful place in your imagination where you can *feel so safe … feel so comfortable … feel so relaxed.*

So I'm going to count from 10 to 1 and as I count you can take some steps towards this wonderful place and by the time I get to 1 … you will be standing right inside … and you can look around you and … notice some of the things that make it just *such a good place for you to be* … so ready now.

10 … I don't know if your mind knows where you're going yet … 9 … but your feet can know as they lead you there … 8 … 7 … they know a place to *feel happy* … 6 … that's right … a place to feel safe … 5 … and I think you'll find it will be light and bright … and nobody else can go in there unless you specially ask them to … 4 … it's a place where you can use your inner mind to daydream … 3 … and when you daydream in this special way … 2 … *your special* … inner mind can *find brilliant ways to do things so you can feel more and more comfortable inside* … nearly there … that's it … 1 … so have a good look around you and notice some of the things that make it just *such a good place for you to be.*

Induction Script: Pretend the chair has turned into a spaceship

Age range: approximately 5–8 years

Just sitting here in the chair (Child's Name) I'd like you to show me how brilliant your imagination is/how good you are at pretending because mummy said you were fantastic at pretending/imagining … If you are the same as me … you'll probably find you can *imagine/pretend better when your eyes are closed* … try it and see … and whichever you choose … eyes open or … *eyes closed will be perfect for you* … so I wonder if you can *pretend right now* that … as *you are relaxing right down* into the chair … and *getting more and more comfortable* … that the chair has turned into a spaceship … and that it's getting ready for take off … listen to the rockets firing … and feel the power as it lifts off … you are at the controls and the spaceship is zooming higher and higher … speeding right up into the sky … and as it goes higher and higher … can you notice your body feeling more and more relaxed … and lighter and lighter as it flies high up above the clouds in the sky … that's right.

Induction Script: Look at the light switch

Age range: approximately 8 years upward

If the child closes his or her eyes, that's great. However, if the child keeps them open, providing a focus will ensure that his or her gaze is fixed on something neutral.

> Settle yourself in the chair and find the most comfortable position for you to listen … and as you do … I want you to focus on that light switch over there … and as you listen and as you focus totally on that light switch … I'd like you to observe whether it becomes fuzzy and blurred or whether the outline becomes more and more defined … and while you're deciding whether *it's fuzzy and blurred* or *the outline gets more and more defined* … I'm wondering whether your eyelids feel really, really light … or whether they *feel really, really heavy* … or indeed whether they will *become even heavier and heavier* … so heavy in fact that they will *want to close straightaway* or whether that will just happen in a little while … or not at all … as *your focus becomes more and more intense* and your amazing mind is more and more focused on accepting all the helpful suggestions you told me you *really want to follow right now* so whether you *let your eyes close … easily and naturally …* to *become even more comfortable …* or whether you try hard to keep them open for a little bit longer really doesn't matter at all … whichever you choose will be perfect for you … so long as you *feel very, very comfortable, comfortable in yourself, comfortable about yourself in every way*.

Induction Script: Comfortable cushions

Age range: any age, with appropriate adaptations to vocabulary

This script assumes that there are cushions in the chair.

> You can choose (Child's Name) whether you want to keep your eyes open as you *relax and listen to my voice* or whether you want to *let them close* so you can *listen* more comfortably and as you *let them close* you will probably *find that a rather nice sleepy feeling seems to start in your eyelids* and I don't know whether that is before or after you begin to *notice a rather nice feeling of snuggling/settling down into the chair* … feeling the cushions underneath you … holding you up/propping you up/supporting you … and as you *sink down into those cushions* can you notice how that feels against your arms and legs … all soft and squashy … soft and squashy and silky/smooth/velvety/furry as you

touch them with your fingers … and as you touch them with your fingers … can you *feel the sensation of the calm and confidence* already beginning to pass into your fingertips … spread into your fingers and up into your arms … and up into your shoulders … and up into your neck and head … and then down again … right down into your chest … down into your tummy … all the way down into your legs … and your feet … so nice to relax and feel the cushions holding you up/supporting you/propping you up like cushions full of calm and confidence … confidence … all around you … spreading into you … this is a nice way to *let calm and confident feelings replace those unwanted feelings* you told me about, don't you think … sinking deeper and deeper into the cushions and down into the chair … *more and more comfortable* with each word I speak … and as you *become more and more comfortable* … it *becomes easier to drift and dream*.

Chapter Three

Ego Strengthening and Self-esteem

Low self-esteem underlies many problem behaviours; for example some children have low self-esteem and try to make themselves feel better through bullying behaviour and by making other children feel bad. Conversely, low self-esteem is also the *result* of many problem behaviours; for example children who are verbally bullied can eventually begin to believe that what is being said must be true. Why, these children reason, would they continually be on the receiving end of such mean and nasty remarks if there wasn't some truth in them? They begin either to doubt themselves, or berate and belittle themselves for not having the strength to stand up to the bully. Either way, self-esteem can plummet.

Problems such as bedwetting or soiling will undoubtedly have a detrimental effect on a child's self-esteem. These children look in the mirror and see someone who is childish, dirty, smelly, stupid or troublesome (no matter how parents try to guard against this conclusion). Where parents are less than enlightened and blame or tease their children who wet or soil, the effect on self-esteem can be devastating.

Self-concept and Self-esteem

It is useful to draw a distinction between self-concept and self-esteem; self-concept is the view or image we have of ourselves, and self-esteem is the value or respect that we place on that image. Thus, children may have an accurate concept or image of themselves, for example, that they are intelligent and bright academically or that they are good at playing an instrument, but if they do not place any value on that concept, esteem can still be low. A child's self-esteem is not always based on the achievements that adults value, for example, a boy may genuinely shrug off being good at math(s) whereas being chosen to be on a team in a casual football game may be highly valued. Geldard and Geldard (1997) have a useful section on self-esteem building in their book *Counselling Children*. Failure to understand the distinction between self-esteem and self-concept can explain why parents and teachers sometimes find it very hard to understand why a child who is academically able does not necessarily have the high self-esteem they would expect him or her to have. There is little point in hypnosis practitioners merely extolling the virtues of an achievement or an image that is not respected. One thing we can try to do is to reframe that achievement or self-image so that the child can see a value in it. And I know this is easy to say, but not always easy to do!

Of course, we also need to remember that not everybody is an achiever academically, artistically or in the sports arena but we shouldn't have to 'achieve' or 'shine' to be loved or respected. Sometimes children feel that they are not loved or valued because they fail to meet their parents' high expectations or because they are unfavourably compared to siblings. As all therapists are aware, these feelings can persist and continue to undermine people well into adulthood and even old age. Appreciation of children's personal attributes is important and acknowledgement of these qualities along with genuine praise will reinforce the good qualities or desired behaviours and teach children to respect themselves as well. The following scripts can be useful in helping children feel loved for who they are and not just what they can do: 'You are very special' and 'Be good at being yourself'.

Sometimes, for whatever reason, children just seem to be unaware of their own personal qualities, often comparing themselves unfavourably with others and thinking they have little to offer. One way of dealing with this is to find out what they value in their friends; this can usually give you a clue as to what other people probably like about them. Your task then is to persuade the children with whom you are working to notice these qualities in themselves since they have already told you that they value them. The following script may be useful: 'You are a good friend'.

At other times, children just need to hear some really positive feedback to let them know they are valued. Hearing a genuine compliment, particularly in a trance state, can have an immensely positive effect. The following scripts may be helpful: 'Compliments' and

'You are a good friend'. When working with children, or indeed working with anybody, it is important to get the balance and credibility right; paying someone an insincere and unfounded compliment will, at best, be ineffective and at worst, destroy the person's faith in you. However, commenting on the fact that you admire someone for trying hard to get over a problem, or giving the client credit for every bit of increased coping or learning ability that has been shown so far will be extraordinarily helpful. Also, acknowledging how well clients are carrying out the hypnosis and how creative their imaginations are sets a good tone; after all, you are the expert on hypnosis and therefore your opinion will be respected. A bit of genuine praise goes a long way, and I always try to encourage parents to do this at home too, trying not to sound 'preachy' or 'condescending' when I suggest it!

On occasion, parents can get so worn down by their child's particular challenging behaviour that all a child hears is negative feedback, which further diminishes self-esteem and can perpetuate the problem; indeed, such criticism might have been part of the problem in the first place. Asking a parent in the child's presence to tell you something that he or she really likes or values about the child can be one of the most useful interventions you will find. It is encouraging for the child to hear something good and it helps the parent to change the focus from negative to positive. This is discussed more in Chapter 12, which focuses on behaviour problems. When a child has been brought to see you partly because of behaviour problems, a useful intervention is to find a way to reframe the inappropriate behaviour so that the child begins to understand that the behaviour has been getting in the way of his or her feeling good.

An encouraging family environment is vital in building a child's self-esteem because the child who has high self-esteem is more able to deal with outside pressure notably that of his or her peer group. The influence of the peer group cannot be overestimated. Individuals with high self-esteem are more able to form their own judgments rather than constantly needing to seek the approval of others. Children who don't fit in with the ethos of the group can have a hard time at school. They can become overly submissive in order to please others and lose a sense of self in the process; they can become lonely and isolated; or be more prone to bullying, feeling disliked and unworthy. On the other side, they can become overly dominant or, at worst, aggressive and bullying themselves. Children with high self-esteem are less likely to doubt themselves and their positive self-concept can remain intact despite not feeling that they are exactly the same as everybody else.

The issues surrounding self-esteem building can be quite complex, but sometimes even complex problems can be helped by taking simple measures such as using an ego-strengthening script, particularly if it is recorded so it can be listened to regularly. There is no doubt that children (and adults too, of course) thrive on being respected, valued and loved and, whatever the reason for their coming to see me, I will include some degree of ego strengthening in the treatment session. There are several scripts of varying lengths to choose from in this chapter and, of course, you can select relevant extracts as appropriate. Sometimes it seems all that is necessary is to incorporate a confidence-boosting phrase or two in the general treatment, whereas at other times the whole session may be built around raising the child's self-image. Reassuring children that they are loved (clearly you need to be sensitive to their circumstances) and telling them something positive that someone significant has said about them can have an excellent effect.

The following scripts are intended for general confidence building:

- 'Ladder of confidence' is a general confidence-building script making use of past positive experiences and positive comments that you elicit in a pre-induction talk.

- 'STOP messages on your mind computer' is helpful for children who tend to put themselves down (perhaps because they have internalised negative messages from other people in the past) or are loath to try new things.

Summary

- Low self-esteem can be the cause or the consequence of prob-lems.
- A self-concept is the view or image we have of ourselves.
- Self-esteem is based on the value we place on the image we have of ourselves.
- Children with high self-esteem are less dependent on constant approval from others and are more resilient in the face of nega-tive peer pressure.
- Children may have an inaccurate self-concept, e.g., they per-ceive themselves as being stupid instead of having difficulties because they are Dyslexic.
- The therapist may want to:
  - help children form a more accurate view of their self-concept;
  - alert them to positive qualities they possess;
  - show them how to value and respect those qualities;
  - remind them that they are loved and appreciated;
  - build their confidence and resilience;
  - pay a genuine compliment whenever possible.

Self-esteem Script: You are very special

Age range: approximately 5–9 years

Do you know (Child's Name), there is nobody else who is exactly *like you …* which means that *you are very special, very special indeed …* so, you can *be very proud of yourself …* just for being you … a very nice person to be … you can feel good about who you are … always remember your mummy/daddy/ grandma/etc. love you very much ☞ **NB Select very carefully here. Choose people who are important to the child and don't make assumptions; grandparents may be dead or the child may not see one parent if there has been a divorce.** ☞ You make them very happy just because you are you … they like the kind and thoughtful things you do and say … they like seeing you *grow more and more confident/brave/happy each day*.

You are growing stronger and stronger and happier and happier … you can *wake up in the morning feeling happy …* you can *enjoy every moment of your day …* and when it's bedtime, you feel sleepy and safe … you're happy to *drift off to sleep …* you *feel safe and happy*, happy and comfy … knowing you can wake up in the morning and *enjoy your day …* you like being you because you're a good person to be … You're a happy and loving person … each day you are learning to *enjoy things a little bit more than before …* enjoy your home, your school, your class and being in the playground too … and each day you can enjoy it a little bit more.

And *do* remember (Child's Name), that *you are a very special person* … there is nobody else who is exactly *like you…* which means that *you are very special*, very special indeed … so, you can *be very proud of yourself* … just for being you … a very nice person to be … always remember your mummy/daddy/ grandma/etc. love you very much … you make them very happy just because you are you.

Self-esteem Script: Be good at being yourself

Age range: approximately 6–12 years

(Newborn babies don't have to be good at things; they're just good at being themselves.)

Have you ever looked at a newborn baby? … A tiny little thing who hasn't yet learned to be good at math(s) or good at sports or good at drawing … they aren't really very good at anything at all yet … but their mum and dad love them with all their hearts … they just look at them and love them because they are their own little son or daughter … already they have their own little personality … which is different from anybody else's … a little person you can love just because they are themselves … they're just good at being themselves.

As you *are good at being yourself* … you have grown a bit older of course … a lot older really … and *naturally you have learned to be good at a lot of things now* … and of course *they are proud of you for all the things you're good at* … and yet … *most of all* your *mum and dad love you because you are yourself* … of course … they think *you're great* because you can do this and you can do that … but most of all … *they love you just because you are you … a very special person indeed.*

Self-esteem script: Compliments

Age range: any age if you adapt the vocabulary

This script requires the parents to do some preliminary work for you. You will coach them on the phone about what you need from them. Their task is to collect a genuine compliment from members of the family or other significant people for you to use within the session. Generally, the comment should be about the child's nature rather than his or her appearance and you should be certain that the comment would be appreciated. It is better not to say anything if you are at all unsure about this because you are also giving the child the suggestion that he or she will always remember it. If you can record this for the child to take home, the intervention will be even more effective. If not, you might provide a written record of it to read at home.

> And (Child's Name) while you are relaxing so comfortably and so calmly here in the chair … just listening to the sound of my voice … I want you to know that your memory has been getting better and better and then when you hear what I'm going to tell you in a moment … it will store these things inside you where *you can always remember them* … so they will be there for you to *remember very clearly* … whenever you need to *feel good about you* … now, I have been collecting some very valuable comments about you from some people who know you very well … I would like you to take each comment and store it very safely in the inner part of your memory … so listen very carefully indeed.
>
> Grandpa said that (Child's Name) is a girl/boy who …
>
> Aunty Claire told me that she loves (Child's Name) because …
>
> Mr Jones said that one of the things he particularly respects about (Child's Name) is …
>
> Uncle Joe says that one very special thing he always remembers about (Child's Name) is …
>
> Your teacher, Mrs Smith, says that something that really impresses her about (Child's Name) is …
>
> Your mum said that she thinks that one of your nicest qualities … and it was hard to choose … because there are so many … is …
>
> Your dad said that he really appreciates your …
>
> So (Child's Name) isn't it good to know that people who know you best think so highly of you and isn't it even better to know that your memory is so brilliant that it will keep all of these thoughts for you to remember every day.

Self-esteem Script: You are a good friend

Age range: approximately 7/8 years upward

Only choose this script if you have checked that the child has at least one good friend and elicit the friend's name beforehand. You can repeat the activity with other good friends if appropriate.

Have the child drift off to a favourite place or use the 'Find the right place' induction script in Chapter 2.

You know how … when we have a good friend … we tend to *notice the nice things about them* … notice *their good qualities* … I'd like you to notice right now that one of your best friends is sitting right here beside you … I wonder what it is that makes you really like this friend … what are the things that make him/her an especially good friend to you?

And now I'd like you to do something a bit unusual … I'd like the part of you that is particularly good at noticing things … to float up … and then float down inside your friend (Joe) for a couple of minutes … so you can be inside your friend (Joe) who appreciates the good things about you and you can know just what those good things are … that's it … nod your head when you're there.

☜ **If the child has any difficulty with this, just explain that he or she can pretend to do it in any way that feels okay.** ☞

And just being inside (Joe) for a moment or two and looking at (Child's Name) … I'd like you to notice what it is that (Joe) really likes about you (Child's Name) …

☜ **Use a selection of the questions below or any others that you think would be useful and relevant. You can get the child to tell you aloud or just to do it internally as you think best.** ☞

What is it that (Joe) likes/admires about/values in (Child's Name)?

Does (Child's Name) make (Joe) laugh?

Does (Child's Name) make (Joe) feel good about himself?

Does (Child's Name) stick up for (Joe) if he needs him to?

Is (Child's Name) loyal/trustworthy/kind?

Can (Joe) rely on (Child's Name)?

Can (Child's Name) be kind/supportive?

And having found out all those interesting pieces of information I think it's time for you to float back up now and float right back down into yourself (Child's Name) … make sure you're right back inside yourself …and feel your own hands and feet wriggling around … and I wonder how it feels to know just how your friend really appreciates you … let yourself really enjoy those feelings right this moment … mmm … understand that these are very good qualities that you have and you can let them grow stronger each day … notice yourself naturally being all of those things that make you such a good friend to be … and noticing too that other people enjoy those qualities in you. As the days and the weeks and the months go by you will notice that you are generally feeling more confident … feeling more at ease with being yourself and being altogether happier in so many ways.

☞ Whether you choose to reorient the child back immediately or include a further script first, be sure to do a lively 'awakening' since you have done a double dissociation here: first, by having the child drift off to a favourite place and, second, by having the child float into the friend. ☜

Self-esteem Script: Ladder of confidence

Age range: approximately 8–12 years

Adjusting the vocabulary and scenarios, this script works well with teenagers and adults too.

It is important that in your introductory talk you elicit positive reference experiences to include in this script, and you need to choose instances that are meaningful to and valued by the child in question. You can also add in positive comments made by parents and other significant people in the child's life. You may have elicited these in front of the child or on the telephone beforehand or both. The script might not be suitable for use where there is a fear of heights but, as safeguards have been included in the script, this may not in practice be a problem. Examples have been provided to suggest the type of experience to elicit from the child.

> And noticing that you are feeling more comfortable and more relaxed now … you are doing it so well … and it's good to know that when you are more relaxed it means you are brilliant/very creative at using your imagination … I'd like you imagine that you can see a ladder up against a wall in front of you … it's a very strong ladder (with handles to hold on to as you go up) and it is fastened to the wall so it is very, very safe … this is your ladder of confidence … and in a moment when I ask you … you are going to climb up the ladder … each step is going to help you feel more confident than before … because with each step you will be remembering some very positive/happy feelings … and when you get to the top, you will be feeling very strong/confident and happy/proud indeed … there are 10 steps on the ladder and each step has got something special … that will help you feel a bit more confident than before.
>
> Let's have a look at the first step … and as you put your foot on it you begin to remember that time when (your teacher told you what a brilliant reader you are/got you to read out your story because it was best in the class) … can you *feel that strong, proud feeling spreading all over you?* … And when *you can really feel it*, you are ready to take the next step up … just nod your head and let me know when you're ready … good (Child's Name) … you *are* doing really well … so, get ready for the thought/memory/feeling as you *carefully place your foot on step 2* … hey, does that feel good? … Do you remember when you scored that goal/your Dad told you how proud he was of you/you got all your spellings right? … *Feel how good you feel inside …* Don't you want a bit more of that strong confident feeling? … Go on, double it now! … Great! Now get ready to go on up to the next step, number 3 … can you guess what you're

going to find/remember up there? … Let's see if you were right … it's when your teacher admired your drawing/you were really pleased with the model you made/passed your exam … fantastic … *get a feel of that confidence* … isn't it good?

⮎ **Continue up the steps in a similar vein, including visual (V), auditory (A) and kinaesthetic (K) expressions. There is of course nothing sacrosanct about the number 10; you could make it 5 steps for a very young child with not a lot of patience! Once you reach the last step, you can continue as follows.** ⮌

Hey, you're amazing. You've done so well … Run/float/jump down to the ground and quickly run up the steps again reminding yourself of just how fantastic it feels each time you stand on a step … remember to take the fantastic feeling from each step with you as you climb up to the next one.

⮎ **Give the child a reminder as he or she goes up again of each occasion and feeling previously linked to the steps, e.g., 'the excited, proud feeling when you scored the goal'. In NLP terms, you are 'stacking anchors'. After you have reached the top of the wall with all the positive feelings in place, you can talk the child through the new scenarios making sure to include VAK modalities.** ⮌

When you get to the top, you can climb over the wall into tomorrow/next week/ your future … look at you (Child's Name) … so strong/brave/confident/proud … *Isn't your face happy and smiling as you are making new friends/are talking to other children? … you've got a real spring in your step as you go to school … listen to your voice as you sound so happy*/really keen to put your hand up in class … how exciting for you to do all those things so easily that once you used to be a bit worried about … how cool is that! … Brilliant! Amazing! Well done! … I want you to know that as each day goes by all of these things become easier and easier, more and more natural to you… *I wonder if it will surprise you or if it will just feel perfectly natural that you are so confident now.*

Self-esteem Script: Wash off harmful messages from the walls of your inner mind

Age range: approximately 10 years upward

I wonder if you can *use your imagination right now* … and imagine that the air around you is a wonderful colour that reminds you of every positive and confident feeling or thought you've ever had … I wonder what colour that would be? … And with each breath you take … *see it filling your body … hear it filling your mind with positive and confident thoughts and feelings* … that's right, the colour spreading all around now as you begin to remember some of *the things that you are good at* … some of the things that you enjoy … was it when you kicked a ball, or played some sport … or sang or danced, or played and listened to music that you love? ... Or maybe you helped a friend, or are thoughtful and loving to friends and family ... maybe you are brilliant about being kind and getting on with people ... do you know that some of the most successful adults are the ones who were not the best at school but they were absolutely brilliant at getting on with people? ... All of these things are very valuable indeed ... just as YOU are very valuable indeed ... so keep breathing in this happy confident colour that reminds you of your strengths and positive resources and let it *spread all around you now* ... and you know you don't even have to *focus on your own positive qualities and abilities* because your own memory will remind you of them more and more each day.

Now *look a little more closely* ... can you *notice any other areas that have a different colour*? ... The colour of any possible tension ... or the colour of self-doubt perhaps? ... I wonder what colours those would be. ... well, if there are any ... begin to *breathe those colours out of your body* ... right out of your mind, *breathe out that tension ... breathe out that self-doubt ...* and *breathe in that wonderful happy, confident feeling* ... and let it *spread all around your body and mind* ... that's right, that's brilliant ... you can do this whenever you want to *feel rather more calm and confident ...* and in this comfortable, slightly dreamy state I want to talk to you about your mind, which is so incredibly clever.

We all have two parts of our mind ... the part we use actively all day to think and talk and work things out ... and we call that our conscious mind ... and we all have another part of our mind we call our unconscious mind (or our inner mind) ... that stores information and knowledge ... stores all our memories, stores our feelings about ourselves and stores our habits too ... I know that *you are very creative and imaginative* and you can *use that excellent imagination of yours right now...* to think about *your unconscious* like a room in your mind ... this is the room where we first developed our beliefs about ourselves and our abilities ... it's a room where we keep all kinds of useful memories, positive opinions, feelings and habits ... maybe we store them in mental cupboards or drawers or even have them written on the walls ... but you know sometimes we store stuff in there that *isn't* helpful ... maybe *unhelpful* negative opinions or beliefs about ourselves which can stop us being the strong confident people we really are meant to *be confident...* we really *are* meant to *be confident.*

Sometimes we've heard somebody else's opinion or belief about us which is quite mistaken, sometimes because they really didn't understand us ... could even have been a silly joke ... could be that we misunderstood what they meant ... something that wasn't meant but we believed it at the time ... It could have come from anywhere ... someone you know or someone you hardly know ... another child, a family member, or even a teacher ... but for whatever reason they had the wrong idea about you.

I want you to know that *those messages are very mistaken and not at all help-ful ...* so I want you to go into your special room in your mind now and look for mistaken, unhelpful beliefs and messages about yourself that are written on the walls ... for example, some people find messages that read ... 'I can't do that, I'm not clever enough'…(or sometimes even worse words like 'stupid') … believe me, they are very mistaken messages and extremely damaging messages … so I want you right now this minute to *wash off any negative message immediately, scrub it right off.*

Now get a paintbrush and dip it in the confident paint right there … and paint that wonderful bright confident colour all over the walls … good, excellent. Wasn't that satisfying? … Of course the important thing now is to program your way of thinking in a positive way … put up new messages on the walls so you get into the habit of … *thinking positively about yourself … think positively about yourself …* write some very positive messages … do it in bright colours and in good strong clear writing … *I am bright … I already have many strengths and from now on I will remember these strengths … I believe in myself … I am a good person.*

Good. Very well done … how about adding three more positive messages for yourself now? … Make them very positive indeed … keep writing … keep programming … ♋ **If you feel the child needs more reinforcement, you can get him or her to open all the drawers and cupboards and check for positive messages. Provide ego strengthening as you think appropriate, but also leave time for the child to put his or her own messages in. Finally, have the child visualise him or herself in everyday situations with positive internal messages and beliefs and notice the difference in the way he or she thinks, feels and acts.** ♋

Self-esteem script: STOP messages on your mind computer

Age range: approximately 12 years upward (possibly younger if they are keen computer users)

The script uses some ideas from cognitive therapy, e.g., thought-stopping and replacing negative thoughts with positive ones. This framework is used again in Chapter 9 to stop obsessive thoughts.

A useful way to think about our brains is that they are rather like computers only far more impressive … so I want you to imagine right now that *you can* … go into your mind computer and click on the confidence program … can you see the confidence window come up? … That's right … now (Child's Name) just have a look and see if it is running properly … sometimes what happens is that there are little error messages in there that need clearing out … for example, some people find messages that tell them ♋ **Be cautious about how you use your voice here so it doesn't come across as an embedded command.** ♋ that they can't do things because they aren't clever enough … you told me that you had that voice in your head that stopped you from doing things, didn't you? … now I want you to *understand that that message is extremely* *damaging* … and *it is a very mistaken message* … so I want you to click on the delete button and *clear that message immediately* … good, excellent. Wasn't that satisfying? … The next thing to do is to set a reminder message so that … if ever that silly thought were to come into your head again … a big stop sign will come up in your mind … it's a big red sign with STOP written on it … can you see it? Make it bright, bright red … make it very big indeed … and listen, it has a very loud voice like this … STOP! THIS IS AN ERROR MESSAGE FROM YOUR CONFIDENCE PROGRAM … and then you remember that *you can do it* … *you (Child's Name) are definitely clever enough* … you are more than clever enough … now type a new message in place of that mistaken one … *I am intelligent and I can learn new things very well … I can learn to be more confident each day* … hear how good that sounds … get a feel of that confidence … isn't it great? … Now before you finish, go and have a look for any other possible error messages … or any other silly, mistaken message that may be spoiling your confidence program. ☞ **Refer to anything that the child may have told you about in your pre-trance discussion.** ☞ Delete everything that is not useful or is harmful to you and type in something that will make your confidence program work better, for example … *I am a positive person, I am calm and I am confident… I can learn new things* … add any positive message that's right for you and now save that information and close the confidence window … nod your head when you've done it … ☞ **Pause long enough for the child to do this. Watch the child's fingers for movements as he or she types the positive messages.** ☞ Now your brain can run your confidence program and each day as you *practise doing everything calmly and confidently* … *you increase your confidence daily.* ☞ **Have the child visualise being in normal everyday situations with his or her confidence program error-free and working properly.** ☞

Useful Compliments and Self-esteem Suggestions to Include in a Script

- I'd like to congratulate you for trying so hard to overcome this problem for it shows you have two great qualities: good judgment and determination.

- You can be proud of yourself for the progress you have made so far. I know your mum/dad is very proud of you and I am very proud of you too.

- I would be proud to have a son/daughter like you.

- You're doing a great/fantastic/amazing job of …

- Your mum and dad love you because you are yourself … a great person to be.

- We all have different parts of ourselves, the strong parts, the confident parts and the shy parts … and sometimes the shy/under-confident parts need a bit of encouragement from some of the other parts that know how to *be confident* … so right now … mentally, silently in your head … please ask the confident part of you to tell the shy/nervous/under-confident part something nice about it … something encouraging … remind that part of something nice about them so they can feel really good about themselves … that's right … you can feel really good about being you.

- You are doing so well at this hypnosis … not everybody can do it as well as you, you know … you seem to have a special talent.

- You have got a brilliant imagination so I know you can do an amazing job of this.

- Each breath you take can remind you of a kind thought you had/thoughtful thing you did/time when you helped your grandma/you stood up for your friend/you managed to cheer up your little brother.

Beginning to Reframe

But now you stop and REALLY think about it (the implication being that it wasn't properly thought about before) perhaps it may seem to you that …

And I can perhaps understand how it USED TO seem to you that it was no big deal to be so good at math(s) but I wonder whether … now you are able to look at it from a more sophisticated point of view you can *find another way to appreciate it*.

It's interesting that you should tell me that being good at drawing isn't important because I had a boy here the other day who told me that it was the one thing in his life that he was really proud of … would you tell him that he's wrong to feel that way?

So, I've heard that the (bullying/unkind/silly) behaviour only really started when you got in with that new crowd of people. I suspect … and I think you might *agree with me* that … that way of behaving wasn't actually right for who you really are. It was more of a mistake that you could *put right now by putting an end to it* so you can then *be proud of yourself for making the right decision* and get back to being your real self … what a relief to be yourself again!

So you're telling me that you spend a lot of time imagining that you aren't good enough … even though that seems to contradict what other people think about you … you know that is really good for me to hear because it shows what a brilliant imagination you have and if you have a good imagination you will be amazingly good at hypnosis … you just need to learn to *use your imagination in a more helpful way.*

I know you like to be thoughtful and helpful to your family so it's excellent to know that you have that part of you that will know just how to be thoughtful and helpful to the part of you that needs some reassurance right now … I'm going to ask that amazingly thoughtful, helpful part of you to remind the under-confident part of you of some very good qualities that you might have forgotten about till now.

I have heard from your dad that you are very protective, very kind and polite to your brothers and your friends so I am amazed to hear how very rude and unkind you have been to yourself … refusing to acknowledge those nice qualities you have … not giving yourself any credit for your achievements … so I think it is time to stop being so rude and unkind and give yourself a break … start being a bit kinder and at least more polite to yourself … give yourself the odd bit of praise … and you can, can you not … start right now … here this minute … by thinking of three very good qualities you possess and politely give yourself a bit of a pat on the back … that's right.

And can you explain to me exactly how 'being shy' means 'being stupid'?

And I wonder if you have ever thought that being a bit shy can you give you a real insight into helping other people feel at their ease?

And interestingly, some people might think it was rather arrogant to refuse to believe it when your teacher/friend/mum/dad say that you are a very valuable member of the class/you're a very nice person to know … and you told me earlier that the last thing you would want to be was arrogant.

Chapter Four

Nocturnal Enuresis

Definitions

Enuresis

Enuresis comes from the Greek word meaning 'to make water'. This chapter focuses on the treatment of nocturnal enuresis, which refers to the unintentional passing of urine during sleep at night, more commonly known as bedwetting.

Primary Enuresis

The child has never been consistently (for a period of about 6 months) dry at night.

Secondary Enuresis

The child has been consistently dry at night for a prolonged period and then begins to wet the bed.

Common Contributory Causes of Nocturnal Enuresis

Slow Development of Regulatory Systems

In primary enuresis the problem is very often due to slow development of the regulatory system that allows the bladder to gradually distend over many hours without emptying. The body is slow in producing enough of the hormone called Antidiuretic Hormone

(ADH), sometimes called Vasopressin. ADH limits the production of urine, particularly during sleep. This slow development can be hereditary so it is not unusual to find that a parent also used to wet the bed after reaching toddler age. If both parents had the problem, it is even more likely to occur in their child.

Small Functional Bladder Capacity

Functional bladder capacity is the amount of urine that can be held in the bladder before feeling a strong urge to urinate. When functional capacity is small, there is a strong urge to pass urine even though the bladder itself may be of normal size and may not be full. In this case children may often need to use the toilet more frequently and urgently during the daytime than their peers and they may wet several times during the night. All of this may be caused by developmental delay but can also be compounded by over-frequent emptying of the bladder during the day.

Physical Problem

Bedwetting can be a sign of an underlying medical problem, such as urinary infection, diabetes, kidney disease or a congenital abnormality of the urinary tract although this is fairly rare. In these cases, you might often (although not always) expect to find difficulties with bladder function in the daytime as well as at night. Just to rule out the possibility of organic problems, always ensure that the parent has checked things out with the medical practitioner before treating the child with hypnotherapy.

Emotional Stress

In secondary nocturnal enuresis, where children have been dry at night for some time before starting to wet the bed, it is probable that there is some underlying emotional stress or anxiety. Nevertheless, a medical problem, such as a urinary infection, is also possible and so, once again, a visit to the medical practitioner is strongly advised.

Common background issues in cases of anxiety include: a new baby, problems at school, upset in a friendship, bullying, family difficulties, death of a family member or friend or even a pet, a house or school move. In fact, anything that disrupts the child's emotional stability can be the cause of or an exacerbating factor in bedwetting and it is worth bearing in mind that a child can be deeply upset by something such as an argument with a friend that an adult might think has no significance at all.

Habit and Mindset

Whether the original cause is emotional or developmental, I believe that habit and mindset play important parts in perpetuating bedwetting and this is where treatment with hypnosis can be particularly focused. The body gets into the habit of relaxing all the muscles in sleep and not noticing and not responding to signals that the bladder is full; this is particularly so in the case of deep sleepers and many mothers report that their bedwetting children are very deep sleepers. Children who have had the problem for many years go to sleep with the mindset that this is a problem over which they have no control and their expectation is that they will wet the bed. Additionally, if they wear protective pants the body is kept comfortably warm and dry and this reinforces the lack of need to control the bladder. It is essential for the body to learn the difference between wet and dry and, generally speaking, I will only agree to treat children when their parents will agree to protect the bed rather than the child.

Deep Sleep

Most of the parents of bedwetting children report that their children sleep very deeply. One of the things I hear frequently is that enuresis alarms, activated by the child wetting the bed, wake everyone in the household except for the child, who, of course, sleeps through the entire event. Even so, there is evidence that enuresis alarms can be effective in some cases, especially when compared to no treatment at all.

Conventional Treatment

Desmopressin (sometimes called DDAVP) is a commonly pre-scribed drug that mimics the natural hormone ADH, which the child may be lacking. The drug's effect is to concentrate the urine and reduce the volume of urine produced. It comes in tablet or nasal spray form (nasal spray has been discontinued in some countries), and although this drug is usually well tolerated, headaches, stomach upsets and nausea have occasionally been reported.

Imipramine Hydrochloride is a drug that is used to reduce bladder irritability. It is also used for adults as an antidepressant. This drug is generally well tolerated but possible side effects include dry mouth, nervousness, sleeping difficulties, fatigue, digestive problems and constipation. Imipramine is less often prescribed because of the risk of side effects. Although these side effects are still fairly unlikely, they are more prevalent than when compared to Desmopressin. Both drugs are thought to improve the situation in about 70% of cases, but improvement does not mean cure: apparently only about 50% become dry during treatment and often the bedwetting reoccurs when drugs are stopped.

Generally speaking, if the drugs are going to work, they will work very quickly. If they do not do so, the dosage may be increased or it may be determined that the child is not a candidate for this treatment approach.

Bedwetting alarms are another frequently used approach. There are various types of alarms, but they all involve a sensor that activates an alarm the moment it gets wet – as the child begins to urinate. The theory is that over time the child will wake before he or she begins to wet the bed, and, therefore, before the alarm is sounded. As mentioned, although there is evidence for the effectiveness of this method, one of the dangers is that the child will sleep through while the rest of the family are awake! In some countries these devices are available for rent or are loaned out free of charge. There are many brands for sale but they tend to be quite expensive.

The parents who bring their children for hypnotherapy are those who do not want to give their children drugs or who have found them to be ineffective for their particular child. Although I have not conducted a clinical trial, the children I have seen have nearly always had a positive outcome with hypnosis and their parents are very pleased to have found an answer that is natural and safe. I must emphasise that children need to have been medically checked to rule out organic problems, that parents need to support the treatment (see below), and that the child's environment needs to be safe and secure. Always remember that wetting the bed is a natural response to abuse of any kind.

Pre-session Talk with Parents

I prefer to ask for certain information out of earshot of the child so I talk at some length with the parent beforehand to discover the attitude of the parents, find out something of the family dynamics that may have a bearing on the child's state of mind and to describe the treatment and ask for the parents' cooperation in supporting the treatment. I explain about protecting the mattress rather than having the child wear protective pants in bed and about the need to be positive in looking for and noticing signs of progress. For example, a first sign of change may be that the child wakes as he or she is urinating and, if this has never happened before, it can indicate substantial progress. A parent who is not alerted to this perspective might understand such an occurrence simply as a continuation of the wetting process. It is important to ask parents never to use the awful phrase, 'He's gone back to square one' if there is a relapse. Such an expression is guaranteed to destroy the child's confidence and undo a lot of really good work. I explain that I will be asking many of the same questions again during the session but I will be talking directly to the child rather than talking to the parent *about* the child. It is very useful to explain tactfully that the session works best when the parents let you take the initiative in inviting them to join in the discussion from time to time rather than their jumping in too quickly to help their child answer questions.

Before and during the session, play detective: try to discover any pattern that may be related to the bedwetting. Find out whether, for example, there are more or fewer wet beds if there has been a difficulty at school, if one parent rather than the other has bed duty or if bedtime is set earlier or later. Find out the pattern of wetting – does it occur at night or the early morning? Does it happen once or more often? The more information you have, the easier for you to know the next step.

Summary

Elicit background facts either before or during the session

- How old is the child?
- Is there a family history of nocturnal enuresis?
- Has the child been checked out medically?
- Are there wetting or urgency problems in the day as well as at night?
- Is there a known cause?
- Is it a long-term problem or sudden onset?
- Has the child ever had a dry night?
- Has the child ever had a month of consecutive dry nights?
- Is he or she taking medication? What are the effects?
- Does the child wear night-time protection?
- What other remedies have been tried? What was the response?
- Are there family background difficulties/marital problems/any other known problems in the child's life?
- What is the attitude of other family members?
- Which factors, if any, make it worse/make it better?
- What will be the best thing about being dry?

Parental role/Tips for parents

- Get the cooperation of both parents to support the treatment.
- Limit drinks after dinner but ensure that the child drinks plenty during the day.
- Eliminate fizzy drinks or drinks containing caffeine, as they stimulate the bladder.
- Limit sugary food; in some children, it also seems to stimulate the bladder.
- Protect the bed not the child (the body has to distinguish between wet and dry).
- Talk of more dry beds not fewer wet beds.
- Unobtrusively, give extra positive attention to the child when the bed is dry.
- Never blame or (worse) punish the child; it is not his or her fault.
- Try not to make an issue of it; the child will be at least as disturbed by it as you are even if he or she doesn't show it.

- Understand that the treatment is a process and while some children have instant results after one session, the likelihood is that progress will take a few weeks (maybe longer).
- Small relapses are normal if the child is ill, overtired or upset; never utter the dreaded words 'Back to square one', which can undo all positive achievements.
- Encourage the child to share some responsibility for bed change if old enough, but never let him or her think of this as a punishment.
- Boost the child's self-esteem whenever possible.

Referral to a Medical Practitioner Before Treatment

Although it is worth repeating that it is important to ensure that the parents have checked with the medical practitioner that there is no organic problem, the likelihood is that they will already have done so. Very often they have been down the route of bed alarms and medication (or they wish to avoid having their child take drugs) with little success and they have come for hypnotherapy as 'a last resort'.

Suitable Aims for Hypnotherapy Treatment

- Change a negative mindset and increase positivity and optimism.

- Build self-esteem and confidence.

- Install the belief that the child can take unconscious control over the problem.

- Increase the child's ability to cope with minor setbacks and understand that the body is learning a new process and a new habit.

- Encourage the child to stick to better drinking habits (as discussed earlier).

- Notice and respond appropriately to signals from the bladder.

- Sleep more lightly and wake when necessary.

- Wake and walk to the toilet (do not use the phrase 'go to the toilet' since many children understand it simply to mean urinate, so it might be misconstrued to mean wake and urinate right then and there in the bed).

- Deal with emotional issues if relevant.

- Deal with stressful situations more easily and calmly.

Things to Bear in Mind

- Always include ego strengthening and praise any progress, however small.

- Always use suggestions and scripts that emphasise the idea of taking and manipulating control. Any of the scripts in other chapters that use ideas of computers and master control rooms may be adapted and applied here as well.

- Always use guided visualisation of the child carrying out the desired behaviour bringing in all the senses – visual, auditory and kinaesthetic (VAK).

- Teach children their homework while they are in trance and get them to visualise it in detail, e.g., every night before they go to sleep spend 2 minutes programming the brain and bladder/visualise themselves getting up and walking to the toilet when they need to go/setting their mental alarm clock to wake at relevant time.

- Before they leave your session ask them to run through any procedures they have agreed to carry out and reaffirm their commitment to these, e.g., bedtime/daytime routines/daily visualisation or listening to a hypnotherapy CD. Getting them to tell you is far more effective than your telling them!

Nocturnal Enuresis Script: Stay dry all night long

Age range: approximately 5/6–9 years

Verify that the child understands the word bladder before you start and use the same words that he or she uses, e.g., wee, pee, go to the toilet, go to the bathroom. It is possible to use this script as a basic framework for even younger children if you shorten and simplify it.

> I'd like you to imagine (Child's Name) a funny thing … that you can see inside your body now … and pretend to see into your tummy … and in your tummy there is the bladder that holds all the wee inside your body … hey, look at your bladder and notice what colour it is … make it brighter and brighter with each breath you breathe in … now notice the door that keeps the entrance/opening to the bladder closed … and see what colour the door is … make sure that the door is very, very strong because it has a very important job to do … it is going to *keep the door closed* … and only open it when you say it can … so, now (Child's Name) put a guard on duty, make sure it is a guard who is very responsible and that the guard will stay awake all the time you are asleep … this is a guard from your special dreaming mind … that special part of your mind which is always awake and looking after you even when your body is fast asleep … you know, it's that part of you that keeps your heart pumping blood around your body and your lungs breathing in the air around you … without your ever having to tell it to do it for you … it just does it because it knows how to look after you (Child's Name) and keep you safe … and … now that we are asking it to … it will help keep the door to your bladder firmly locked at night when you go to bed … so you can *stay dry all night long* … *stay dry all the way through.*

> Now make sure that the guard has the key … is it a big key? What colour is it? … Of course you must go to the toilet just before you lock it up … And then *lock it up tightly after you have had a wee*/after you have emptied your bladder in the loo … and if you want to … you can even bring in another guard to make sure *that door stays tightly shut all night through* … now, tell that guard exactly what to do if your bladder gets too full in the night … as soon as it feels the signal from your bladder that it's full up … it must call out loudly to you 'Wake up, (Child's Name) … Wake up' … And when you *do wake up* … you must *get up and walk to the toilet* where you can *empty all the wee from your bladder down the toilet* where it all belongs … then you will *feel so pleased* … and immediately tired again … that you go straight back to bed and go fast asleep … as soon as your head touches the pillow.

> Now, of course sometimes your bladder won't be really full up … and then the guard's job is to … *keep that door tightly shut all night through until morning* … all *through the night tightly shut* … *keep your bladder tightly shut* … Either way, when you wake in the morning … your bed is dry … your night clothes are dry … you feel warm and dry and happy … *you feel great because you know that you are in control … you are in charge of the wee … you have taken*

53

complete charge of your bladder ... and *you can keep it tightly closed all night through* ... notice the happy feeling inside you ... you go downstairs and speak to everyone ... they notice that big happy smile on your face ... and you tell them that ... yes, the bed is dry ... great! Well done. *You (Child's Name) are in control* ... look at their faces too ... they've got big smiles too.

You know, all day you feel great, strong, confident and well rested because you got all your sleep last night didn't you? ... And, you know what? ... Each day and each night this quickly becomes your normal habit ... and I don't know how soon it will be ... before there are *only* dry nights ... at first, it may be one or two, and then three or four nights ... or it may be that from this time on *you only have dry beds* ... each day *you feel happier and happier* ... *you feel more and more confident and relaxed* ... you know that *your special* mind is able to ... *keep your bladder tightly shut* ... and if you need to get up to go to the loo, it will shout loudly ... 'Wake up' ... Then you will *notice it instantly* and *get up and walk to the toilet* ... and have a *wee in the toilet* where it really belongs.

Have a look now at the picture on your imaginary television ... it's you (Child's Name) ... each day you make sure that you drink a lot of water during the day ... see yourself at teatime having your last drink of water ... look at you at bedtime making sure the very last thing you do is to go to the toilet ... and look at you so comfy in your bed ... Just imagining very carefully locking up the door to the bladder and making sure the guard is on duty ... remember that your special guard will shout out loudly the exact moment it can ... *feel any signal from your bladder* so you ... *get up, walk to the bathroom* and have a wee in the toilet where it belongs ... then see yourself waking in the morning to a nice warm dry bed ... just look at that happy face (Child's Name) as you realise your bed is dry ... you are dry, you feel fantastic and so proud of yourself ... you are in charge of your body now ... brilliant. Well done!

Nocturnal Enuresis Script: Wake up and get up when you need the toilet

Age range: approximately 9 years upward

Maybe you can imagine now that you have an album of photos of you and your life ... and now can you turn back the pages to you when you were younger? ... Can you see a picture of you when you were about 5? ... What did you look like when you were 5, I wonder? ... Now find one when you were very young ... when you were very, very little and you were learning to walk and you used to fall down sometimes as your *body was learning this new skill* ... can you see now a photo of you falling down ... and then another one of you just *picking yourself up again* ... of course it was no time at all before you could walk easily ... *take things in your stride easily* ... because this is what children do ... their *bodies learn a new skill* and then they *just do it naturally* ... *easily* ... after a bit of *practice* ... and if you turn over the pages in the album that show you growing older ... you can see yourself having learned to do all kinds of things that once seemed hard but now with a bit of practice can *seem so natural and easy to you.*

I'm sure you know that professional athletes/footballers/dancers practise to get things exactly right … but did you know that they not only practise in the gym/on the football field/dance floor? They spend a lot of time with their trainers practising everything in great detail in their minds first and then their mind helps their feet get it right … helps their body get it right … because the mind is the part of you that sends all the tiny little signals to the body to *use this muscle or clench that muscle to make sure the right thing happens in the body at the right time in the right place.*

So right now your amazing mind can do a bit of practice, just like the athletes/footballers/dancers, to help *your body do the right thing … in the right place … at the right time too* … I'd like you to use your mind to program your body to *clench all its bladder muscles to … keep your bladder closed when you go to bed … so your bladder stays tightly closed when you are in your bed …* first of all … mentally, silently send this message to your bladder muscles right now so they know you *really* mean it and nod your head when you've done it … here goes … '*stay tightly closed when I'm in bed all night long*' … that's it … now see a picture of you completely warm and dry in your bed when you are fast asleep and still in complete control … nod your head when you can see it … great … now send another message to your bladder to *send a very strong signal when it is full* and it needs you to *wake up* … make it a very clear message so it knows just what to do so *you are in time to wake up and get up* … nod your head when you've done it … now see a picture of you fast asleep but just noticing a feeling somewhere in your body … yes, even when you are asleep … that lets you know your bladder is full and you need to *wake up … get up… and walk to the toilet …* nod your head when you can see it.

Now see the picture of you when you get up and you are walking to the toilet in the middle of the night … *you only use the toilet* … you *never use the bed* because you *only do things in the right way at the right time and in the right place now* … nod your head when you can see it … great … that's right.

Now see the picture of you when you have emptied your bladder/had a wee/had a pee in the toilet and you are walking back to your bed in the middle of the night … you only use the toilet … you *never use the bed* because you *only do things in the right way at the right time and in the right place now* … nod your head when you can see it … great … that's right … this is how you practise … you are doing this so well.

And just as those athletes and those footballers and dancers practise again and again to get it exactly right … we're going to get some more practice too … nod your head when you are ready. ☞ **Repeat the steps above of the seeing him or herself waking up and getting up and walking to the toilet several more times, getting quicker and quicker each time. Include practice of the child seeing him or herself getting up again later in the**

night (or very early morning if this is the pattern of wetting that has been established in the pre-induction talk). ☞

Wonderful … now I would like you to see yourself climbing back into bed and immediately drifting back to sleep calmly and comfortably and feeling very pleased with yourself and very pleased with your body for being able to carry out all your instructions and wake you up to get up whenever you need to empty your bladder … nod your head when you can see this picture … great.

Now very quickly I'd like you to go through all of that one more time before we finish … just as though you are there now … step into the picture and be there now and feel yourself climbing into bed and remembering to send your programming messages to your bladder … program your body to *clench all its bladder muscles to … keep your bladder closed when you go to bed … so your bladder stays tightly closed when you are in your bed* … now program your bladder to send a strong signal to wake you up when it is full so *you are in time to wake up and get up and walk to the toilet* … you only use the toilet … you never use the bed because you *only do things in the right way at the right time and in the right place now.*

Excellent. Well done. In a few moments I'm going get you to come back to the room but just before we do … remember that photo album? … I want you to put two photos in there … first put a photo of that old bedwetting habit back in the place where you keep all those old habits you have grown out of … remember the ones … crawling instead of walking/sucking your thumb/falling off your bike? … Great this photo belongs with them … belongs to long, long ago.

Now put the new photo in the today section of your album … the one of you and your dry bed habit with your ability to program your body to *keep your bed dry* … make sure you look good and are smiling for the camera! And when you've done it you will notice that you *feel lighter and brighter all over* … all the energy is coming back into your hands and your fingers … wanting to wriggle about … wanting to stretch perhaps … you will already *notice yourself feeling more confident* and that *confidence will increase every day* … not only about your ability to *control your bladder all night long* but in every area of your life too … at home … at school … out and about … wherever you are … filled with an inner confidence so that you take everything in your stride.

Nocturnal Enuresis Script: Calm and stretch your bladder

Age range: from about 8 years upward.

Adapt the vocabulary as necessary. This script is for use with a child who has been diagnosed with small functional capacity and possibly an irritable bladder too. Usually there will be urgency and frequency problems to some extent in the daytime as well as at night-time. You can also insert relevant parts of this script into any other script you are using.

It seems that your bladder has been a little bit *over*sensitive … it's been trying to do a very good job at keeping you comfortable but it's been overdoing
things a bit … so you are emptying your bladder a little more often than is really
convenient … especially at night … so let's ask it to *calm down now and give
you a bit of peace and quiet* … and it's good to know that here and now in this
pleasantly day-dreamy state *your very special* … inner mind is particularly open
to ideas that will help you *feel better … feel calmer and feel more comfortable*
all over your body … *feel calmer all through your body.*

So let's program your mind/get your mind … to send some messages to your
bladder … I'll tell you what to say and you can say it silently in your head … you
can use your own words if you want to … ready? … Bladder, please calm right
down … ☞ **Pause long enough after each phrase for the child to repeat
it mentally.** ☞ there's really no need to be *over*sensitive any more … you can
stay cool/calm/relaxed and take things a bit more easily … you can *stop over-
reacting* … have a bit more confidence in yourself … know that you can *stay
calm, comfortable and in control* even if there is quite a lot of liquid … *you can
hold on* until it's convenient to go to the toilet.

Well done. Perhaps you can see a picture/image in your mind now of your bladder looking calm and relaxed instead of being oversensitive … I wonder what
that would look like? … I wonder what calm and peaceful colour it is?

Now we know, of course, that you have been getting a little older and your
body has been growing more mature every day … and *you are able to do so
many things now* that you didn't know how to do when you were younger …
and one of the things that your body has been learning to do is to *stretch its
bladder and hold on to that liquid/urine/wee inside for a longer and longer time
… yes … stretch itself and hold on for longer and longer* and now you have told
it exactly what to do/programmed your bladder … what you need is a bit more
practice (Child's Name) at that stretching and being able to *wait more calmly
and easily* before you need to go to the toilet …

One way to get that practice is to just imagine yourself in every situation where
you would like to hold on a bit longer … holding on easily and effortlessly …
waiting far longer than you thought you could, couldn't you? … that's it … see
yourself at home watching the television holding on a little bit longer and a little
bit longer because your bladder is stretching and the muscles are tightly closed
… great … keep the muscles tightly closed and know that you can let your
bladder fill up a little bit more and a little bit more … yes, there's plenty of room
… of course you're doing it brilliantly … *notice how comfortable you can feel
while you are waiting* … how normal it can feel to *wait calmly and just know
deep down inside that you can wait even longer still … you are in control* …
you can let your bladder fill up a little more and a little more each day … really
imagine exactly how good that feels right now … notice how your bladder can
feel so calm while it's waiting … ☞ **Depending on the child's age and tolerance, run through visualisations of as many everyday situations as you
can at home/at school/out and about/in the car.** ☞

57

And as *all the nerves in your bladder become more and more calm* in the day-time and *you are waiting longer to let your bladder fill right up* before it needs to empty …. you will find that *at night-time too you are taking more and more control … your bladder nerves are so much calmer than before … your bladder can stretch and hold on for longer and longer while you sleep …* every night when you go to bed I want you to remember to send that message to calm the nerves in your bladder so they stay calm and comfortable … the bladder stays closed tight and allows it to fill right up with all the muscles keeping it completely closed.

Then I want you to set the alarm clock of your bladder so that the bladder *stays firmly closed while you are asleep* and … if you really need to go … it will begin to ring and ring and ring so loudly that it wakes you up in time to *get up and walk to the toilet* … set it right now for practice … turn the alarm hand round and round until you see the words 'time to wake up … I need to get up and go to the toilet' … and then click it into place so that … if you *really* need to go … it will *begin to ring and ring and ring* so loudly in your head that it wakes you up in time to *get up and walk to the toilet.*

Now just before we finish I want you to practise all of that in your mind so that you can see yourself getting into bed … snuggling down … sending all the messages from your mind to your bladder … that's it … look how you are really concentrating on it … notice yourself noticing all those calm feelings now your bladder has calmed down and has just stopped being oversensitive … see how you are setting your bladder alarm to wake you when the bladder is really full … and just see yourself now asleep … feeling really comfortable and calm … that's right … your bladder muscles calm and tightly closed all the time you are asleep in your bed … your mental alarm clock will ring loudly if you need to get up and go to the toilet … brilliant … amazing … well done.

And now it is time to come back to the room with me feeling very positive, very happy and completely sure/confident that your body is learning new habits really, really well … you are completely sure that you will *remember to program your bladder and set the mental bladder alarm every night when you go to bed* … all the energy is coming back into your hands and your fingers … wanting to wriggle about … wanting to stretch perhaps … you will already notice yourself feeling more confident and that confidence will increase every day … not only about your ability to *stretch your bladder all day and all night long* but confident in every area of your life too … at home … at school … out and about … wherever you are … filled with an inner confidence so that you take everything in your stride.

Chapter Five

Encopresis

Definitions

Encopresis

Encopresis is the term used to describe the process of soiling underwear or passing faeces in inappropriate places, usually after the time when children have previously been able to control their bowel movements. It usually occurs around or after the age of 4 years old. Faecal soiling is normally involuntary and associated with constipation, but occasionally it can be deliberate. Before treating a child with regard to soiling, it is essential to refer the parent to a medical practitioner to rule out any possible organic problem.

Primary Encopresis

Soiling that has occurred since birth, suggestive of an organic problem.

Secondary Encopresis

Soiling that occurs after a child has had bowel control for at least 6 months.

Constipation

Infrequent and/or painful bowel movements caused by faeces/stools/poo moving slowly through the intestines so that the waste matter becomes harder or pellet-like and thus more difficult to pass without discomfort or straining. Although there is a wide variation in normal individual frequency, the term infrequent typically refers to 3 or fewer times per week.

Faecal Incontinence

The passage of bowel movements without awareness, or the inability to prevent the passage of a bowel movement.

Faecal Impaction

A large mass of hard faeces stuck in the rectum caused by continued stool holding and severe constipation, normally requiring removal by a medical professional.

Possible Signs of Constipation

- Infrequent bowel movements.
- Painful bowel movements.
- Reluctance to use the toilet because of the expectation of pain.
- Soiling that may be runny, often referred to as leakage, over-spill or seepage.
- Vague, or at times, severe abdominal pain.
- Decreased appetite, nausea, vomiting.
- Lethargy, irritability.
- Night-time or daytime wetting caused by pressure on the bladder.

Referral to a Medical Practitioner Before Treatment

It is relatively uncommon to find an organic cause of constipation in young children. Nevertheless it should always be ruled out by a medical practitioner before you make that assumption. Even if, as is most probable, the problem is found to have no organic cause, the constipation itself needs to be addressed by a clinician to clear out the colon. Hypnotherapy can then be very effective for reducing fears, installing and then maintaining new habits.

Possible signs indicating a need for investigation may include:

- episodes of constipation of more than 3 weeks.
- the child is unable to take part in normal activities.
- small, painful tears appear in the skin around the anus.
- the appearance of haemorrhoids around the anus.
- stool is not expelled through normal pushing.
- involuntary leakage of liquid or runny faeces.

Incidence

Encopresis is likely to occur more frequently in boys than in girls. Evidence suggests it occurs in 1–3% of children under the age of 10 years old. It appears to be independent of social class and does not seem to run in families.

Pre-session Talk with Parents

The most common cause of overflow soiling is constipation, so this should routinely be investigated before assuming that the soiling has a psychological origin. Parents are sometimes, understandably, loath to consider that constipation could be the cause of the problem since the faeces can be runny and very frequent and so the pattern seems to contradict the generally accepted view of constipation. Sometimes, if the stools have been very loose, a mistaken diagnosis of diarrhoea may even have been made and medication to 'dry up' diarrhoea may have been used, which will, of course, have exacerbated the problem. In order to avoid potential embarrassment to the child, it is useful to gain as much information as you can before the session with regard to the causes of soiling and probable constipation. During the session itself you can then be more selective in your questions. (A list of common causes follows.)

Generally speaking, soiling is involuntary and it causes children to feel embarrassed or awkward. The older the child, the more this is true and the greater the loss of self-esteem associated. Blaming and punishment can only make the situation worse. Tactful discussion of this before the session can help to ensure that your efforts are not undermined at home by parents or siblings. Deliberate soiling without accompanying stool holding is thought to be quite rare and could be suggestive of emotional disturbance and is sometimes found in children with Conduct Disorder or Oppositional Defiant Disorder. This is then best dealt with alongside professionals specialising in these areas. Family therapy can be particularly helpful.

Suitable Aims for Hypnotherapy Treatment

I will deal primarily with the area of 'soiling associated with constipation' since it is far more common and is the one that is likely to present in the consulting room. Although constipation is the cause of the soiling, emotional problems such as low self-esteem, anxiety and embarrassment may well be a consequence, and these conditions can be treated with hypnosis once medical/lifestyle treatment of the constipation is underway. Treatment will almost certainly include something to soften the stool to make its passing easier and more comfortable for the child so that you can truthfully suggest that 'doing a poo will be easier now'. Looking at the causes of constipation itself can help us decide which suggestions are relevant to include in a particular child's treatment.

Some of the Common Contributory Causes of Constipation

* Diet lacking in fruit, vegetables and other fibre.
* Diet with *excessive* milk, sugar, wheat, protein and refined products.
* Not enough liquids, particularly water.
* Lack of exercise (compounded by the lethargy that results from constipation).
* Ignoring the urge to have a bowel movement.
* A previous painful experience on the loo.
* Changes in life or routines.
* Certain medications.

- Over-enthusiastic toilet training.
- Emotional stress such as a new baby, death in the family, bullying, marital or family disharmony.

Ignoring the urge to go to the toilet can arise for many reasons and when you find the likely ones it is important to include coping strategies for them in your hypnotic suggestions. It can be something relatively simple, for example, that the child doesn't want to be interrupted when playing with toys or watching a television programme, or is embarrassed to ask where the toilet is when in somebody else's home, or is embarrassed to go because the parent is not there to help him or her clean up afterwards. Embarrassment can start very early in some children and shouldn't be underestimated. The same can be said about anxiety. Anxiety about strange toilets or dirty or smelly toilets can cause some children to get into the habit of withholding at school or nursery school/kindergarten, and it doesn't take much for this withholding habit to turn into a constipation problem. Some children are worried about spending time in the toilets at school because they come to realise that this is where bullies often hang out. Small children may have fears about falling into the toilet itself or about snakes, rats or monsters living there – ideas that may have been suggested by siblings, friends, or television programmes, or that are simply products of a vivid imagination.

Consequences of Constipation May Include Both Physical and Emotional Aspects

- The stool is hard and painful to pass and so the child avoids the repetition of pain by withholding, thus increasing the likelihood of pain and withholding occurring again.

- As a consequence of frequent overload of the bowel, rectal muscles become overactive, which conversely causes the anal muscles to relax. The internal muscles continue working to try to eliminate (unsuccessfully) the mass of collected faeces. This forces the very soft or liquid faeces to bypass the blockage and continue down the rectum to the anus where the relaxed anal muscles just allow the seepage to occur quite involuntarily.

- The child gets dirty, may smell, becomes embarrassed and gets teased, blamed or even punished for doing something naughty whereas, in reality, the issue is probably totally outside his or her control. All of this, of course, can be quite distressing and self-esteem can plummet as a result.

Reviewing the above can help us to choose which of the next suggestions may be appropriate, assuming that a dietary or medical treatment for constipation is being followed. Whichever suggestions you select, use the child's preferred language according to age and family culture, e.g., 'push that poo right out of your bottom' or 'push the waste matter right out of your body'.

Hypnotic Suggestions and Interventions

- Self-esteem and ego strengthening.

- Release or reduce anxiety or phobic reactions.

- Notice the feelings in the child's tummy telling him or her that they are signals that he or she wants to go to the toilet.

- As soon as the child notices the feeling, he or she walks/runs to the bathroom and pushes it out into the toilet where it belongs. (NB Don't use the phrase, *'go to the toilet'* because for many children this is merely an instruction to defecate and they may respond to the suggestion literally, right then and there!)

- Doing a poo/going to the toilet/having a bowel movement will be easy/fun/different/satisfying from now on.

- Enjoy using the toilet/enjoy the sensation of pushing the stools/poo out of the body.

- Feel so much better afterwards.

- Enjoy taking control of their body/taking charge of their poo.

- Breathe in through the nose and out through the mouth while pushing (holding the breath inhibits easy elimination) (push not strain).

- Drink water and eat as instructed by the medical or nutritional practitioner (normally plenty of fibre in cereals, fruit and vegetables).

- Sit on the toilet after a meal for 5 minutes since this is a natural time for elimination to occur. Read a comic.

- Deal with accidents as appropriate and as agreed (parents: don't turn cleaning up into a punishment).

- Reinforce any instructions from the medical practitioner, having first checked that the child understands what has to be done.

Emotional Problems and the Impact on the Bowel

There is plenty of anecdotal evidence to suggest that emotions affect the workings of the bowel in both adults and children. Those who suffer from Irritable Bowel Syndrome (IBS) are well aware of the effects of stress and tension on their condition, so interventions aimed at relieving anxiety and tension and increasing feelings of emotional security will almost certainly be helpful when treating children who present with 'toilet difficulties' of any kind.

Small children who have been too enthusiastically toilet trained may associate bowel movements with stress, anxiety, frustration, blame or angry feelings (both their own or their parents' responses) and may subsequently develop withholding behaviour in an effort to avoid the tension of the 'toilet experience' or possibly even at the unconscious level to frustrate their parents' wishes. Struggling with parents for control may cause some children to hold stools back as long as possible. It would be particularly useful with such children to include the suggestion that they are very much in charge of when, where and how they do a poo and that every time they sit on the toilet they get a strong feeling of being in charge. The 'Poo in the toilet' script could be suitable in such a case as it begins with the imagery of painting out negative feelings or worries. Very often young children will 'paint' with their hands as they act this out in their imagination. Indeed it could be wise with very anxious children simply to concentrate on a worry-release intervention plus ego strengthening in a first session and only to introduce the toilet aspect at a second meeting. Several short sessions at frequent intervals for the very young are far preferable to a long drawn out one every now and again, and if you have the facility to record some self-esteem building suggestions onto CD, this makes ideal home listening as they go to sleep at night.*

We need to remember that where there is severe constipation, stool impaction and consequent soiling, hypnotherapy on its own will not solve the problem no matter what the original cause. The colon needs to be cleared out under medical supervision. Ideally, hypnotherapy can be given in order to allay fears prior to any physical intervention whether this is through laxatives, enema or physical removal. After colon clearing, hypnotherapy will be very helpful indeed in alleviating emotional distress and helping to install and then maintain more appropriate, regular toilet habits. Where it seems that the original problem was an emotional response to harsh toilet training or to blame and punishment for accidents, the parents will need to be tactfully encouraged to change their attitude or the chances of recurrence will be high.

Apparently Deliberate Soiling or Smearing

As suggested above this is a problem that has presented in my consulting room comparatively rarely and has nothing to do with constipation. This deliberate act of passing of stools in inappropriate places seems to have an emotional or psychological cause where there are issues of rebellion, control and/or where there may be dysfunctional family relationships. It may be that children who manifest the behaviour should be referred to professionals specialising in these kinds of problems, but I have included a couple of scripts that I have used successfully, and that could be tried

---

* Go to www.firstwayforward.com for a wide range of CDs covering common childhood problems.

out first or used in tandem with other approaches. One script is based around indirect suggestions and metaphor so as not to further antagonise the child, 'Right time and place/jigsaw'. Another, 'Mr Smelly Poo' is based on the externalisation approach of White (1989/1997) and White and Epston (1990) and is inspired by their idea of 'Sneaky Poo'.

Where you find that a particular approach or script seems to suit the individual child with whom you are working, you may find it useful to take the framework and construct something similar for subsequent sessions.

Externalisation is a linguistic process where you aim to separate a problem from the person so that the person doesn't feel blamed for having it; in other words it is the behaviour rather than the child that is the problem. There is the criticism that in doing this, children are not required to take responsibility for their actions, but in my experience it is more a way of allowing them to save face and, at the same time, gain their cooperation in finding inventive ways to attack, outwit and, it is hoped, solve the problem. Children can be very defensive about 'being a problem' and clam up if asked questions about it, particularly if there is a history of blame and punishment. 'I don't know' can become a standard answer whereas if you invite them to play detective and help you out in finding ways to outwit the problem, they can be much more forthcoming and creative. There is a wonderful book entitled *Playful Approaches to Serious Problems* (Freeman, Epston & Lobovits, 1997) that illustrates how this process works within the context of narrative therapy with children and their families. Of all the books I have read, this one has influenced me most in my approach to children in the consulting room.

Soiling Script: Poo in the toilet

Age range: approximately 4–6 years

This script could also be shortened and adapted to use just for gentle toilet training with children as young as 2 or 3 years old.

> This is your very own resting story … I wonder if you know how to rest, really rest … I wonder if you could pretend that you are really resting so well that if someone were to look at you they would think you are nearly asleep … I wonder if your arms are all floppy ? (hands/legs/feet, etc.) … It's good to feel comfy and even a bit sleepy as you snuggle down … while you listen … because we all like to feel comfy and safe … and I wonder where you first … begin to feel that gentle warm, comfy sleepy feeling spreading around your body … does it start at the top and go all the way down your body … down to the very tips of your toes? … Or does it seem to spread out from the middle of your tummy … all over all the way through … brilliant … that's right …
>
> I think you are really ready to hear your resting story. It's called The Magic Garden … Can you see you are in a magic garden? … Can you see the green grass under your feet … and feel it under your toes? … Look up, and maybe you can see a fluffy white cloud in the blue sky? … Can you feel the sun, gently warm on your skin? … Oh, look over there … can you see the flowers with wonderful colours … maybe you can even smell them as you walk by? … Listen, they are magic flowers and they can talk … The flowers are saying 'we love you … you're really special … yes, you … you're really special … and because you are special, you can feel very happy'.
>
> Keep walking and then you see there's a little table and chair … look, your chair has got your name on it … great … what colour is it? … Why don't you sit down? … It's just the right size for you … and look … what's on the table? … There are some special pens and paints and paintbrushes and some pieces of drawing paper … do you know what they are for? … They are there for any girl or boy who's got any worry or bad feeling or problem inside that you really don't want any more … some children have problems with wees … and other children have problems with their tempers … but I know you had a bit of a problem with poos … and now you can get rid of your problem … pick up a paintbrush … have you got it? … And begin to paint away your problem onto the paper … paint it right out of you … you can use any colours you like to paint out any bad feelings … paint out any frightened feelings … paint out any sad feelings right out of you … so you can feel light and happy all over … on the inside … on the outside … inside out and all the way through … keep painting till you've left all of that problem behind you … brilliant … that's right … wonderful.
>
> Now you've painted that worry … painted that bad feeling right out of you … how does that feel? Does it feel light and warm inside you now? Well done! … You can feel so good … good on the inside of you … good on the outside of you … inside out … all the way through.

And begin to walk back up the garden path, where you see the flowers again … listen, they're calling out to you … 'Come and touch me' … and the orange one is saying, 'I'm the magic brave and strong flower … when you touch me, you feel so, so brave … touch me and feel how brave you are … you feel all brave and strong all over on the inside, on the outside, inside out' … so touch it now and feel how brave you feel all over inside, outside, inside out. Can you feel it? … That's great.

And then the blue one calls out … 'I'm the magic poo flower and whenever you touch me … you will feel bright and happy … and you will *know how easy it is for you do a poo now* … can you feel that easy feeling going into you when you touch me? … Does it feel a bit like a tingling feeling? … My magic is changing your body so *it's easy to do a poo now* … this special feeling makes you grow stronger and stronger so you can … *be in charge of your body* … that's great … now you've touched me … the blue poo flower … you really *enjoy that great feeling of pushing that poo out of your body … push it out right into the toilet/potty* … great … it feels so good … have a look … there it is … well done … you are so clever … you are in charge all of the time now … so you can keep your pants/knickers nice and clean … you smell so fresh … it's really nice to be near you.'

Look there's a red flower. What is it saying? … 'I'm the magic red flower that can help you *notice feelings that tell you that you want to do a poo …* when you touch me, you can always *notice/feel the feelings in your tummy/bottom* (or anywhere in your body) that tell you it's time to run off to the toilet straightaway. You notice the feeling wherever you are … you notice it if you are playing … after you've been eating … whoever you're with … whatever you're doing … and straightaway … *as soon as you notice that feeling in your tummy … you really want to run off quickly to sit on the toilet and push that poo right out of your bottom/body into the toilet* where it belongs … you do it in the toilet so your pants/knickers stay nice and clean and dry … hey, doesn't that feel good? … You are in charge of your body now … every time you sit on the toilet you can say to yourself … *'I'm in charge of pushing this poo into the toilet'*.

And now you feel so bright and so brave and so strong and so happy you know you can do anything you want to … you know you're happy because you've got a big, big smile on your face … you look a bit like Thomas the Tank Engine when he has a big smile on his face … well done.

☞ **If the child has the tolerance to listen further at this stage, you could include some guided visualisation of their carrying out your suggestions. However, it is better to err on the shorter rather than the longer side and, in any case, the child will doubtless have been visualising it all as you made the suggestions. You can do more on a second visit.** ☜

So every time you come back to your magic garden … you will hear those flowers saying … 'you are so special … we love you' … and then you feel all the happy feelings all over … and your mum/dad/grandma/teacher/dog/elephant loves you too … they are very proud of you … and I think that *you* are very proud of you too … and you can feel happy all over, on the inside, on the outside and inside out.

I think it will soon be time to come out of your magic garden now … and when you do … now … you will have such a lovely day … maybe it's time to have a lovely big stretch now … that's it … and now you can enjoy every single moment of your day.

Soiling Script: Robot help station

Age range: approximately 4–6/7 years

Adapt the gender and description as appropriate to the particular child you are treating.

So I think you are ready to hear your resting story … This is a story about a little boy called (Child's Name) … One day (Child's Name) was watching TV and he decided to watch a DVD called (Child's Name) and the Robots.

Can you see there's a young boy, who looks about 5 or 6 years old and has dark hair and dark brown eyes … He's quite tall and he's wearing jeans, a tee shirt and trainers … ☎ **Describe the clothes the child is wearing.** ☎ This must be your story (Child's name) … so why don't you jump into it now and have a look around you? … Can you see you are in the middle of a green grassy path that leads up to the children's robot help station? … The sun is shining and the sky is blue … Can you see it? … Can you feel the warm sun on your skin as you walk along up to the help station? … And look … can you see all around you there are lots of very special robots? … They're special because all of the robots here have a very special job to do … they help look after children, any children who have worries and problems … Lots of children come to the help station to ask the robots to help them sort out their problems.

'Hello (Child's Name)', said a friendly robot … 'We've heard a lot about you and we know you are a very special boy … and we know you are a very clever boy too and a boy who likes to stay clean and tidy … do you know our job is to help any boy or girl who has any worry … or any problem … or any old habit that they don't want any more? … What you have to do is to walk right over here … that's right … and can you see there are lots of different little tables and chairs with special friendly robots standing next to each of them? … This is where boys and girls have left all kinds of problems and worries and old habits that they're really fed up with … so if you've got anything that you *would like to get rid of* … why don't you walk right over here … some children have problems with wees and other children have problems with their tempers … but I heard you had a bit of a problem with poos … look … the back of your chair has got a balloon on it and it's got your name on it … great … why don't you sit down and look at what's on the table? … There are lots of small robotic toys that are specially for transforming problems … choose the one you want and as you … twist it and turn it … you *twist and turn all the problems out of you* … so you can let them go completely … you just *twist out any bad feelings … twist out any frightened feelings … twist out any sad feelings … right out of you* so you can *feel light and happy all over* … on the inside, on the outside, inside out and all the way through … keep twisting and turning till *you've left all of that problem behind you* … brilliant … that's right.

Well done (Child's Name), said his personal friendly robot … now I'm going to touch you on the shoulder with my robotic arm (Child's Name) … can you *feel the strength going into you*? … Does it *feel a bit like a tingling feeling*? … You are transforming your body into a body that can *find it easy to do a poo now* … this special feeling makes you grow stronger and stronger so you can *be in charge of your body* … (Child's Name) … you can *be in real charge of your body* so you *notice the feelings* that tell you that you want to go to the toilet … you *notice these feelings in your tummy* and *straightaway you really want to rush off … really quickly to… sit on the toilet* and *push that poo right out of your body into the toilet* where it really belongs … and as you push … you *always remember to do a big, big breath out* …a big, big breath out helps the poo *come out really easily* …you *notice the feeling wherever you are* and *as soon as you notice it, you rush to sit on the toilet* and do it in the toilet so your pants stay nice and clean and dry … hey, doesn't that feel good? … Good to *be in charge of your body … you are in charge of your body now* … now you've transformed your body, you really *enjoy that great feeling of pushing that poo out of your body … do a big, big breath out* as you *push it out right into the toilet* … listen to the noise … is it a splosh or a plop? … Great! … It feels so good, doesn't it? … Have a look … yes, there it is … well done … you are so clever! … you are in charge now all of the time so you can *keep your pants nice and clean* and smell fresh and really nice to be near.

You can know you are just like your friends now … you know that whenever you notice those feelings in your tummy, you rush off to the toilet and *enjoy sitting on the toilet* …and as soon as you sit on the toilet, you *enjoy pushing that poo out of your body* … doing a big, big breath out … feeling so good … feeling so special … and feeling so proud that *you have transformed yourself into a really good pooer!* …You *stay clean and dry* because now you just *love doing it in the toilet.*

Sometimes, when you are at school … out and about … or when you're just playing at home with your toys or with your friends … you remember how the amazing robots helped you *take charge of your body* and then you *remember how special you are.*

You always know that mummy and daddy ☙ **as appropriate** ❧ love you so much and when they find out that *you are in charge of your body now* … they will have big smiles on their faces too because they are so proud of you … so every time you come back to your special robot help station in your mind … *all those special happy feelings spread all over you* … you are happy you can

71

feel big and brave and strong and in charge … at home … out and about … wherever you are … you feel so happy … so strong and so much in charge … all over inside, outside, inside out and outside in.

So now I think it's time to say goodbye to the robots for today and jump back out of the DVD so you can open your eyes/feel all the energy flowing back into your body right now … that's right … have a good stretch and welcome back!

Soiling Script: Change your toilet habits

Age range: approximately 8–12 years

This script installs new habits and positive feelings after there has been treatment to relieve the constipation itself.

And having drifted off to this special place where you can *feel very comfortable … feel very comfortable with yourself in every way* … I want you to know that here you can *use your fantastic inner mind to do some amazing things … of course you probably know that it is your inner mind that helps you to breathe even when you aren't thinking about it … helps your heart to beat … helps your skin to heal if you scratch it* … so you can talk to your special inner mind and ask it to help you … *make some wonderful changes* … now that old *constipation problem has been sorted out and your poo/stools can be quite soft* … you can reprogram/fix your toilet habits in just the way you like … you can feel totally comfortable all over … all the way through.

You can talk very quietly in your head so it's only your inner mind that hears you … and I'll give you some ideas of what to say so just nod your head when you are ready to begin … that's right. ☺ **Leave plenty of time for the child to repeat or rephrase your words in his or her mind. You can add encouragements as appropriate.** ☺

- Inner mind, please help me *take control of my body*.

- Help me *notice the signals and feelings in my tummy/body* when I need to go to the toilet.

- As soon as I *notice the feeling* … I will *rush to the bathroom*.

- *As soon as I sit on the seat I will push it out of my body into the toilet* where it belongs.

- Doing a poo/going to the toilet/having a bowel movement will *be easy from now* on because I am eating and drinking the right things … *drink lots and lots of water*.

- Help me to *remember to eat lots of vegetables and fruit so that it gets easier and easier every day*.

- Now I will *enjoy using the toilet/enjoy the feeling of pushing the stools/poo out of the body*.

- Help me to remember to *breathe out through the mouth when I push* because that makes it easier.

Well done … now you have got your inner mind helping you … things *WILL get better and easier every day* …every day you *feel more comfortable and relaxed when using the toilet … each day it gets easier and more and more natural* … it kind of slips out so easily now … so … I wonder how soon it will be before *it is all second nature to you now* … completely, perfectly natural to *do your poos in the toilet … ONLY in the toilet* … whenever you feel the urge … *and you will notice that feeling … you will rush off to the toilet and be really proud of yourself that you are in charge of your body now* … you are in control.

So … two more things to do before we finish …first … I want you to just go back to your inner mind and thank it for helping you *take charge of your new toilet habits* in that brilliant way … … … … well done … and now … let's just zoom forward to the time when … *you have absolutely, completely got over those old problems* … can you see yourself on that television screen in your mind?

Look at you so confident and so pleased with yourself now that *you are in complete control of your body now* … very proud of how you overcame that old problem … well done … and look how proud your mum/dad/etc. is of you … just notice that calm and relaxed look on your face … just see how when you're playing and you get that feeling in your body … you instantly get up and go to the bathroom … as soon as you sit on the toilet seat you feel the urge to push … so you take a deep breath and then *breathe out as you push* … and get that satisfying, slippery feeling as you push that poo/those stools so easily right out of your body … so satisfying … so easy.

And whose idea was it, I wonder, for you to go and sit on the loo and read your comic for 5 minutes after you've eaten … did you just *know that it was a good time for the body to naturally want to do a poo*/expel the waste matter/go to the toilet? … Was it your clever idea or did someone tell you about it? … Brilliant idea … you have done so well … I wonder exactly what the very best thing about it is for you … whatever it is … enjoy it … enjoy being you … a great person to be by the way.

Deliberate Soiling Script: Right time and place jigsaw

Age range: approximately 8–12/14 years

This is a script using an indirect approach to address the problem of deliberate soiling.

This may be the right time for you to take a few minutes to relax and do something just for you ... nobody else but you ... feel good about you ... here in this place ... and there usually *is a right time and a right place for everybody ... a right place for everything* ... a space where you can *think differently* ... a time when you can *see things in a new way* ... when you can *feel more calm and at ease* ... and *things seem to fall into place* ... all on their own.

So let's see if we can *find that place ... find exactly the right place ... for you ...* where you *know what you really want in your life* ... maybe it's a place you know ... a place you've been ... or maybe it's just a wonderful place in your imagination where you can *feel so safe ... feel so comfortable ... feel so relaxed.*

So I'm going to count from 10 to 1 and as I count you can take some steps towards this wonderful place and by the time I get to 1 ... you will be standing right inside ... and you can look around you and ... notice some of the things that make it just *such a good place for you to be* ... so ready now ... 10 ... I don't know if your mind knows where you're going yet ... 9 ... but your feet can know as they lead you there ... 8 ... 7 ... they know a place to *feel happy* ... 6 ... that's right ... a place to *feel safe* ... 5 ... and I think you'll find it will be light and bright ... and nobody else can go in there unless you specially ask them to ... 4 ... it's a place where you can *use your inner mind to daydream* ... 3 ... and when you daydream in this special way ... 2 ... *your special* ... inner mind can *find brilliant ways to do things so you can feel more and more comfortable inside* ... Nearly there ... that's it ... 1 ... so have a good look around you and notice some of the things that make it just *such a good place for you to be.*

One of the reasons *this is a happy place to be* is that ... here and now ... your mind can be especially good at remembering good times ... it can *remember some good times* when you have done something you are proud of ... remember a time when you have had a positive thought ... a thought perhaps that it would be nice to *do something kind* for someone else ... (even if you didn't actually *do it at the time*) ... you were actually able to *think of doing something nice for somebody else* ... all these things can make us *feel happier inside* ... and when we are feeling happier inside it's a good time to think of ways to change some things that we aren't so happy with ... are not so proud of ... things we might do differently ... so we can *feel more comfortable* about who we are and what we do ... *feel proud* of ourselves.

You know you can do this by doing a jigsaw in your mind ... See a jigsaw picture of that soiling/messy/old problem that was making everybody so grumpy and making you so unhappy ... have a good look ... look at how cross and unhappy everybody looks … now can you see (Child's Name) getting into trouble? … Feeling bad? … shouting? … Now see all the other things that don't feel right.

I want you to know that your inner mind is fantastic at doing mental jigsaws and it can *find the answers to all kinds of problems* … so, now please take out all the pieces of the jigsaw that are part of the problem … and ask that special part of you that is so good at doing puzzles in your mind to … take out the troublesome pieces … and find some new pieces to fit in … new pieces that can solve your problems now … find the right shapes … maybe you can see the different pieces now with the right pictures on … so you know just what to do instead … as you daydream now … and even if you can't see exactly what is on the picture … fit in the piece with the right shape and later while you sleep … the new pictures will appear … It can find pictures of (Child's Name) looking calm and happy … altogether more comfortable … so why not have a daydream now … and *begin putting all the right pieces in the right places now* (long pause) … … … or maybe that very clever part of you will fix it all in your sleep … all on its own … and I wonder if it will be a surprise to you tomorrow … when you *notice that all the right bits are in the right places* … just naturally as if it's always been the thing to do … you are acting out all the new parts of the jigsaw … in fact *you're feeling much happier and more comfortable and more confident altogether* … more calm and more confident in yourself … about yourself … all the way through.

I wonder how you just knew that it was the right thing to do to … *feel so much happier and feel so good about yourself* … I wonder who else will *notice all the things that you're doing differently now* your mind has got a new jigsaw picture … It's not only you (Child's Name) but everybody seems to be getting on so much better now … you are so much happier now you are in charge of your feelings … you are in charge of your body … you are in charge of your actions … you are in charge of yourself and you can be very proud of you … well done! … you've done brilliantly, (Child's Name!) … and now I think it's time for you to come back from that special place knowing that tonight while you sleep … your special … inner mind is continuing to sort things out for you … in just the right way … put everything into place in just the right way for you.

So as I count from 1 to 10 you will come back wide, wide awake … not that you've been asleep … feeling absolutely great … so much better and so much more positive and happy in every way … Great … Count up.

75

Deliberate Soiling Script: Mr Smelly Poo

Age range: approximately 5/6–8 years

Before you start, elicit some good ideas the child has had in the past (perhaps writing/telling a story or thinking up a game to play) to which you can refer in the first paragraph of the script (see the first and second lines).

> And as you let your mind drift off to that special place in your mind where you are so good at thinking up new/clever/brilliant ideas … just like when you thought up those stories/imagination games/… you can enjoy letting all your body relax in that comfortable special way you have … just like when you … *go to sleep* … your arms *all floppy and tired* … your hands and your fingers … your legs all *floppy and a bit heavy* … in fact the sleepier your body gets the more your mind can … *dream up some brilliant ideas … to fight back .. find a way to get the better of old Mr Smelly Poo* so he can't make you stink any more … so you *can refuse to let it make you/stop him making you all mucky and uncomfortable* … so just take a moment or two to think up a really good idea to *stop him before he gets started* … and while *your mind is thinking up some really good ideas* … I wonder whether *your body is getting sleepier still … getting sooo sleepy* … getting really good ideas … getting really comfy and relaxed.

> So, let's see … *stop Mr Smelly Poo before he gets started* … I wonder how *you could do that*? I wonder if you can really begin *to notice what is going on* a little while before the poo tries to get out? … I wonder if you could even begin to look for clues to *find out if* smelly poo likes to slip out when you are angry … or when you are tired … or when you are sad … and if *you are a really good* detective … perhaps you could even *beat him at his own game!* … You could notice that if it usually happens when you get really cross … maybe for example, like you told me … when your mum won't let you play on the computer/buy you that game/watch that TV programme/seems to blame you when it's not fair … the very next time it happens that you get some cross feelings … you could *be on the lookout for smelly poo* getting up to his tricks and trying to get you into trouble … you could go and sit on the toilet and beat him at his own game … do your breathing … *breathe the angry feelings out of your mind* with a big out breath … do they have that red colour you told me about? … and *push the poo out into the toilet* before it has a chance to slip out into your pants and muck you up/get you into trouble/make you all smelly.

> So now you have thought up some ideas … let's get you to *see them working really well in your mind's eye … think them through … take all the time you want … watch your own back/catch old smelly poo at his own smelly game/discover a way to stop him from getting you into trouble …*

> And when you're ready you can open your eyes (if they are closed) and tell me which of your ideas is best … or if you don't want to tell me now … you can just see how brilliant you are this week and next time I see you, you can ask me to guess which way you chose to watch your own back and stop his smelly game.

Chapter Six

Tics and Habits

Vocal and Motor Tics

Tics in younger children are normally transient. Estimates are that 1 in 4 children may develop a simple tic during school age that will disappear spontaneously as they get older. Children vary in how much or how little they are affected by them. In some cases it seems to bother the parents far more than it does the child, whereas some children are deeply upset and embarrassed by them. Obviously their environment and the response of other children play an important role here. Tics can be motor (blinks, twitches of mouth, nose or eye) or they can be vocal (grunts, snorts, throat clearing or sniffs). Children can suffer from either vocal or motor tics, or they can suffer from both at the same time and tics can be transient or chronic.

Characteristics of Tics

- Tics can be simple and involve just one or a limited number of muscle groups resulting in a single movement, or they can be complex and involve several muscle groups, which produce sequences of movements, even stereotyped movements such as dancing or jumping.

- They are usually repetitive although irregular.

- They can be mild (usually) or frighteningly forceful.

- They are involuntary although sometimes they can be consciously controlled or suppressed with great effort and associated tension.

- Usually tics disappear during sleep or deep relaxation but sometimes they will persist in light stages of sleep. Sometimes, in fact, they appear in relaxation after periods of activity.

- Tics are generally more prevalent in boys than in girls and more prevalent in children and adolescents than in adults.

- Onset is frequently between 3 and 8 years old although it can occur much later than this and even into adulthood.

Transient Tics

- Transient tics may come and go over a period of months, sometimes one tic replacing another until they gradually decrease and cease altogether.

- They may well be more evident when the child is tired, ill, stressed or excited.

Chronic Tics

- These tics can persist for years either singly or coexisting with several different tics.

- Tics can also often be found in children suffering from ADHD or OCD. Sometimes the medication used to treat ADHD can cause, increase or conversely decrease associated tics.

Tourette Syndrome (TS)

Tourette Syndrome (TS) is a complex neurological disorder that causes multiple motor and vocal tics. It was originally named after Dr Georges Gilles de la Tourette, a French neurologist at the Salpetriere Hospital in Paris who first reported it in the medical literature in the 1880s. In order to be diagnosed as TS the tics will normally have begun in early childhood, or at least before the age of 18, and both vocal and motor tics will have been present and have continued for more than 12 months, although they may be of variable intensity and frequency. Children who suffer from TS frequently have ADHD and OCD symptoms and sometimes self-harming tendencies as well.

Tourette's is often thought of by the general public as the condition in which people can't stop themselves from swearing; in fact, swearing is only one of many aspects that may or may not accompany the disorder. TS can include one or more of the conditions Coprolalia (the uncontrollable use of obscene language), Echolalia (repetition of other people's phrases), Copropraxia (the use of obscene gestures) and Echopraxia (copying of other people's gestures). These patterns can be particularly perplexing and irritating to other people and cause teasing, or worse aggression and physical abuse, because the TS behaviour appears (mistakenly) to be done on purpose to annoy. Swearing and obscenity causes offence and can have difficult consequences for children and their parents to contend with so that, not surprisingly, sufferers often become withdrawn and isolated.

The exact cause of TS isn't yet known, which is also the case with other non-Tourette's tics, but it does seem likely that there is a genetic component that passes on a general disposition towards suffering from it as it tends to run in families. Nevertheless, TS can also occur when there is no evidence of family history and the cause is unknown. It is three to four times more likely to occur in males than females.

Transient tic disorder and chronic tic disorder are on the same spectrum as TS but they differ because the symptoms may not persist or they may not occur so often during the day and there may only be evidence of either motor or vocal tics instead of both.

Medication (Haloperidol, Pimozide, Fluphenazine and Clonidine) may be effective in reducing the tics themselves but it rarely reduces them by more than 50%. With many children the medication has unpleasant side effects (such as excessive sleepiness), although Clonidine is often better tolerated than the others. In certain cases, the side effects are so unpleasant that parents try to get their children to manage without medication if possible.

The term Paediatric Autoimmune Neuropsychiatric Disorders Associated with Streptococcal Infections (PANDAS) is controversially and contentiously used to describe two groups of children; first, those who already have either a tic disorder, Tourette Syndrome or OCD and whose tics, obsessions, and/or compulsions intensify dramatically following streptococcal infections; or second, those children who have no history at all of tics or obsessions and compulsions but who suddenly develop symptoms following a Group A Beta-Hemolytic Streptococcal (GABHS) infection, such as Strep Throat.

Refer to a Medical Practitioner

Refer to a medical practitioner before hypnotherapy treatment to ensure that the problems are not symptoms of a condition that needs further medical investigation. As always, do not lead the parents to believe that you can cure the problem; speak in terms of managing and lessening the severity of the symptoms and building confidence and self-esteem.

Suitable Aims for Hypnotherapy Treatment

- Increase calm and relaxation.
- Build confidence and self-esteem.
- Change perception of the problem so it can be seen as just a part of life that they can cope with rather than feel overwhelmed by it.
- Cope with embarrassment.
- Cope with other people's responses – irritation, frustration, teasing, bullying.
- Encourage them to feel able to explain the problem to others without embarrassment or shame.
- Become aware of signs that the tic is about to occur and install triggers for control of the tic at this stage.
- Take control over the tic for longer periods of time, agreeing on times and places of their choosing to release tension through free expression of their tics.
- Take control over the tic in specific places or on specific occasions.
- Deal with possible related problems such as OCD or ADHD.

Suitable Approaches

- Any focus or relaxation inductions with direct suggestions for calm and control. (Sometimes it is better to bring in the relaxation element only after having focused their attention elsewhere through use of a more visual approach.)
- Include any of the above suggestions that are relevant to the specific child, either directly or indirectly.
- Guided visualisation of successful handling of the problem.
- Any metaphor that allows them to get a sense of control and manipulate symptoms, such as 'master control room' or 'computer'.

Habits

Habits such as thumb or finger sucking and nail biting differ from tics inasmuch as they are, or can easily become, under the conscious control of the child. Even though children may say that they don't know they are doing it, the habit will become conscious when their attention is drawn to it and there is a definite conscious choice whether to stop or continue it at any moment in time. Tics, however, are involuntary, or can only be controlled with a huge effort of will with a great deal of resulting tension. You can expect a habit to respond easily and quickly to suggestion as long as the child in question is truly motivated to stop. Your key task is to discover that motivation, which is sometimes easier said than done! One of the chief obstacles to successful outcome is that it is frequently the parent, as opposed to the child, who has the greater motivation since the habit is most often a source of comfort for the child, which he or she is loath to forego. Therefore, when treating children for a comfort habit, it is clearly crucial to include suggestions for comfort and support in those situations where they might previously have engaged in such a habit. Although most of the scripts in this chapter deal specifically with tics, they can very easily be adapted to reduce or eliminate habits too.

Tics Script: Spaceship master controls

Age range: approximately 5–8 years

Just sitting here in the chair (Child's Name) I'd like you to show me how brilliant your imagination is/how good you are at pretending … because mummy said you were fantastic at pretending/imagining … if you are the same as me … you'll probably find you can imagine/*pretend better when your eyes are closed* … try it and see … and whichever you choose … eyes open or … *eyes closed will be perfect for you* …

So I wonder if you can *pretend right now* that … as *you are relaxing right down* into the chair … and *getting more and more comfortable* … that the chair has turned into a spaceship … and that it's getting ready for take-off … listen to the rockets firing … and feel the power as it lifts off … the captain is at the controls and the spaceship is zooming higher and higher … speeding right up into the sky … and as it goes higher and higher … can you notice your body feeling more and more relaxed? … And getting lighter and lighter as it flies high up above the clouds in the sky … that's right.

And as you go higher and higher into space your body continues to feel lighter and lighter … and any old tight or jerky or shaky unwanted movements are just floating away from your body into a special chute where they are ejected into the sky. ☞ **If the child is very young, you could just float the movements out of the window.** ☞ Your body is getting more and more comfortable … more and more relaxed and calm … all over and all the way through … wonderful … by the way, have you noticed the controls for flying the spacecraft/ship? Aren't they amazing? The captain is asking you to *take charge now* … and make it go a bit faster … and now try it a bit slower, and now change direction. Hey fantastic (Child's Name) … *you are completely in charge! You can slow things right down whenever you want to.*

I want you look right over there (Child's Name) where … because it's your very own spaceship just for you … there are some even more special controls … these are the very special knobs and switches that *calm the feelings in your body right down* and *slow the movements in your body right down* … look over there at that one that looks a bit like a clock … that one's very interesting … it's the special control for making your body calm and relaxed all over … can you see there's an arrow on the clock? … Can you see it over there? … What colour is it I wonder? … When it points to the top, it means that your movements are faster and jerkier but when you *push it right down* … so that it points to the bottom of the clock … you can *slow them right down* … you can *slow right down any tight feelings* and *calm down any shaky movements* and make them *feel calm and relaxed and gentle and almost completely still* … why don't you have a go right now? … I want you to *push that arrow down towards the calm, relaxed feelings* … that's right … give it another push … great … can you *feel those warm, comfortable, calm relaxed feelings* spreading all over your mind and body, on the inside, on the outside, all the way through? … Can you *feel those warm, comfortable, calm relaxed feelings* making you *feel so relaxed* that you *know* you can *be in charge of your body movements any time you want?* ... *And keep them calm and relaxed whenever you want to ... and keep them calm and relaxed wherever you want to ... whoever you're with.*

So now, any time you want to *take complete charge of all the movements in your body ... you can slow them right down* ... so if ever they are too jerky or shaky or twitchy ... you can calm them down by moving the arrow ... you can even make them completely still if you want to ... this control is fantastic ... it can *make all parts of your body behave perfectly* ... just how you want them to ... and *you will feel really great* ... brilliant ... just notice how good it is to *feel that still calm feeling all through your body* ... fantastic ... whenever you want to calm down any movements anywhere just go back to your special control room and push that arrow all the way down ... you're in charge ... well done ... amazing!

But do you know what? ... It's time for you to come back down to earth and land your spaceship now ... steer it all the way back and land it very, very gently ... no bumps at all ... and when you open your eyes you will find that you're sitting here in the chair with me ... and you've been so still that I'm sure now you would like to *have a good stretch* ... to make sure you are wide, wide awake.

Tics Script: You are in charge of your muscles

Age range: approximately 6/7–12 years

Since tics usually diminish while engaging in mental or physical activities, this script builds on children's natural ability to be tic-free while playing football or any other game involving running and a lot of muscular activity. If you intend to change the game from football to another, be sure to read through the script thoroughly in order to adapt sections when necessary.

(Child's Name) I'd like you to let your mind *drift and daydream* and *remember one of those football games* you were telling me about ... I know *you have an amazing imagination* so I'd like you to *be there right now in your mind*/pretend that you are there right now ... playing in the team ... you're wearing your kit ... you can feel the ground under your feet ... is it hard or soft? ... You're playing really well ... and *you're really enjoying yourself* ... notice how you're running and *your muscles move just when you want them to* ... feel your muscles move the way your brain tells them to when you kick the ball ... your feet know just how to *move at the right time* when you pass to your team-mate ... *you are completely in control naturally and easily* as you run up the field ... and as you even think about scoring/saving that goal ... your brain is sending all its precise/clever messages to your muscles to *relax or move in exactly the way that is right for you* ... brilliant ... you are doing this so well ... can you hear the cheering? ... It's wonderful the way *you are naturally completely in charge of your body* as you enjoy the game.

And did you know? … that you can use that natural ability/special part of you to *take charge of your body at other times too* … just as easily … just as naturally as when you're playing football … all you have to do is to let your special imagining mind send all the right messages to your body at the right times for you … so why don't we do that now?

First I want you to imagine there's a football right there on the ground in front of you … but look … it's gone a bit flat/got a puncture and it needs a bit of pumping/blowing up … Why don't you pick up that pump and as you pump the air into the ball … I want you to pump into the ball any unhappy/negative/unwanted thoughts that you might have had so you can *feel so much better without them* … that's right, keep pumping and as the football fills … you will *feel better and better about yourself (Child's Name)* … and you can pump out of your mind and body any out-of-control movements … or unhelpful beliefs about your body … pump out any unhappy thoughts or negative messages about yourself … pump *those old thoughts and feelings away* … right into the football until it's completely blown up … and nod your head when you've finished … wonderful … and what do you think you're going to do now? … That's right you've guessed it … you're going to kick that football as high and as far away as you possibly can … maybe you can kick it so high that you can kick it into that cloud up there? … So the cloud just floats it right over there and far away … far away … or maybe you kick it so far off into the distance … you can watch it floating over people's heads … right over those buildings … right over those trees so all those *old thoughts and unwanted movements never bother you again … they never bother you at all.*

That's brilliant … but there are still one or two things left to do just before we finish … Look up and you will see that there is another football … an amazing golden football up there coming towards you … it's coming towards you in just the right position for you to head it into the goal in front of you … It's coming down towards you and when it touches your head it will *fill you with fantastic feelings of calm and confidence* … here it is … are you ready? … Can you *feel those warm, comfy, calm, relaxed feelings spreading all over your mind and body*? … All over … all the way through … These amazing warm relaxed feelings are sending the message that *you are totally in charge of the muscles in your body/shoulders/arms/face now* … they're sending the message to every part of your mind and body. ☜ **Continue giving specific, positive suggestions about relaxing and controlling the movements that are relevant to the particular child you are treating.** ☞ From now on *your shoulders/mouth/face muscles are going to feel so relaxed and comfortable* … just like *they do right now* … that they only want to move when *you* want them to … they *feel so relaxed and comfortable* that *you are able to take complete charge of those old twitches* and *enjoy letting all of your muscles relax easily and comfortably wherever you are … whenever you want to … you (Child's Name) can take charge of relaxing your muscles wherever you are … whenever you want to … whomever you're with … you can take complete charge of relaxing all your muscles.*

🕮 Another option is to include a time and place, which has been previously discussed with the child, to allow his or her muscles to twitch as much as desired. 🕮

[From now on you will *feel more and more in charge/in control everyday* … any time you want to … when you're at home/in your room/after school … you can let your muscles do whatever they want to do … but whenever *you* choose … you will *take control* … just send a little message to your muscles to say you *want them to relax … stay calm and still* and comfortable … and so they *do stay calm and still and comfortable* at school/when you go out/at your friend's house.]

From now on you will feel so relaxed … so great … and so happy that you can hardly remember how you used to feel … you remember to *forget about those old twitches altogether* now *you are in charge of your body* and you (Child's Name) remember to *feel happier and happier every day* and know that you can do anything you want to *do very calmly indeed.*

In a few moments time you are going to come back to the room with me, feeling absolutely fantastic but just before you do … I'd like you to see a picture of you in your head/in your mind when you're at school/with your friends/in church with all your whole body looking so relaxed and still … 🕮 **Elaborate as appropriate with as much relevant detail as possible.** 🕮 … a big, big smile on your face because you know you can *keep your movements calm, confident and under your control* … your friends/mum and dad/granny and grandpa looking at you and noticing *how happy and relaxed and how still you are … you just look so happy … you feel so happy and you hear a little voice inside reminding you that you are very happy indeed … so, feeling fantastic and knowing that you've done a really good job right here and now … you can open your eyes and enjoy the rest of your day … maybe feeling you want to wriggle your fingers … wriggle your toes and have a good stretch … well done.*

Tics Script: Turn off the tic

Age range: any age

For young children you can make the script very short, and for older ones you can include more relaxation, more repetition and more guided visualisation of positive results.

How about enjoying a bit of relaxing time right now? … You can do it however you like … you can let your eyes stay open or you can *let them get really comfortable* and *let them close right now* … whichever you choose will be perfect for you … you can *let your arms relax first … let them go all floppy and tired* … or you can *let your legs relax first* … it really doesn't matter which way you choose to *relax right now this moment … let your legs relax first* or *let your arms relax first* … because *you are in control/in charge of the way you let all the muscles in your body relax* … And will you *let all those muscles relax all in one go* or will you relax *just one or two at a time?* … *Try it out now* and see which way you prefer … which way is better for *enjoying that relaxing happy feeling all over and all the way through?* … That's right … you're very good at this.

And you can still be finding that out as you listen to my voice that seems to … help you *feel all sleepy and tired* but just awake enough to *do something very clever indeed* … I want you to know that somewhere inside of you there is a place where you can *go inside and find the switch to turn off any tight feelings/tension or any jerky movements* … *in any part of your body* … I don't know whether you have ever done this before or whether *you will be doing it* for the first time and finding out just *how easy it is to turn off the tightness/tension/jerky movements and turn on the relaxation* … so nod your head when *you are ready right now* to *go inside and switch off all the tightness/tension/movements in the muscles in one arm* … all on your own … and *notice how it gets floppier and floppier like a rag doll* … *heavier and heavier as every tiny bit of movement disappears* … *nod your head when you've done it … … …* brilliant … *now nod your head when you've actually done it so well that you can hardly feel it all* … *you can hardly feel it at all* … fantastic … ☙ **Start with arms and legs and then work through the relevant areas in the body. Don't start with facial muscles if that is where the tic occurs. Get the child to turn off some other areas first. You will probably find that the younger they are the quicker they will do it. Don't make the mistake of thinking that speed means they aren't complying; they just do things more easily and quickly than adults do. Look for evidence of limbs relaxing more and more. If your therapy approach includes touch, it is useful to pick up the arm and let it drop heavily into the child's lap. If not, I would advise you against physical contact as it could cause unnecessary misunderstanding. ☙**

It's good to *know that you have learned to turn off those old jerky movements* so well here with me because now you can *turn them off wherever you want to* … *turn them off whenever you want to* … *turn them off when you're with other people* … *turn them off when you're on your own* … and every day *you get better and better at turning them off* … so how soon will it be, I wonder before *there are absolutely no jerky movements* … *no twitches at all* … *you go all through the day every day and you feel absolutely calm and relaxed* … *all through your body/all over your face* … wonderful … you've done this so well … now just before we finish I'd like you to see yourself in your mind's eye/on your mental television screen/on your pretend television when you're at school and you're talking to your friends and … look at you … *you are so relaxed* … *your face looks so happy and relaxed* … *your mouth is all comfy and relaxed* … *your eyes are calm* … *you're smiling and happy and you feel absolutely amazing because* … *of course* … *you are amazing!* … *You are completely in control.* ☙ **Run through all the 'tic scenarios' that the child described in a similar way. Fill them with relevant detail and the names of people who are important. ☙**

And I'm just wondering who is most pleased for you now that you have learned to *turn off all those movements whenever you want to*? … And who is most surprised that they just don't happen any more? Is it mum or dad … your teacher … granny or granddad (as appropriate) or is it you? … Or did you already know deep down that you could *take charge of your body all over and all the way through*? Amazing!

And now I think it's time for you to wriggle your toes and wriggle your feet and have a wonderful stretch as you open your eyes and come wide, wide awake.

Tics Script: Noises or twitches

Age range: approximately 10 years upward

(Child's Name) I'd like you place your hands very, very lightly on your lap with your fingertips just barely touching your legs … that's right … exactly like that … and now concentrate very hard on one hand … I'd like you to *be very patient* as you do this and to *focus all of your attention on the lightness in your fingertips* … I wonder how you could *experience that lightness?* … I'd like you to be so aware of the lightness in your fingers that you can *notice an urge for one of those fingers to move … twitch a little* … that's right … that's amazing … and I'd like you to know that one way that *your amazing* inner/unconscious mind can communicate with you is through little movements in your fingers … little movements that can even *lift your finger* … all of its own accord … that's it … it can *take control* of your finger … to *give you a signal* … let's try it now … I want you to ask your inner mind … just mentally, silently right now … to give your finger a little signal … a little twitch/movement/feeling/sensation/tingle to let you know it is listening … so that when it moves/lifts … *it is telling you it's listening* … brilliant … well done.

So now you know your unconscious mind is very helpful … it showed you it wants to help you by *taking control* of your finger … I'd like you to explain to your unconscious/inner mind … again mentally, silently in your mind … why making these noises has been a problem for you … and why you want to *stop making those sounds* … explain in detail how *it will be so much better for you when you have them under your control* … and nod your head when you've done it … great … ask your inner mind to give you a signal in your finger that it has heard how you feel … great … wonderful (Child's Name).

Now *you* know … and *I* know … that there is a part of you that can already *control those noises at certain times when you concentrate* … and I'd like you to ask your unconscious/inner mind to help that special part of you *get stronger and stronger* and *take charge of those sounds for longer and longer times during the day* … *control those sounds for longer and longer even when you aren't concentrating* … ask your inner mind to *do that now* and *give you the signal in your finger when it agrees* … wonderful … what a fantastic mind you've got

... so please just say thank you to your mind for agreeing to help ... and isn't it good to know that now it really understands that *you want to take control of those sounds* ... it's going to find a way to help you *make these sounds less and less* every day ... and as *it is making these sounds less and less every day* ... it will also *make them quieter and quieter ... less and less ... quieter and quieter ... more and more in control* ... now I don't know *how soon it will be before* these sounds *disappear altogether* but I *do* know that your unconscious mind is very independent and it will *decide to do it in the right way ... in the right time* ... and *in time* for you ... it's about time that *you are feeling happy and positive about you ... you feel really happy and positive about you.*

Now imagine that this is the day (Child's Name) after *the sounds have disappeared altogether* ... see yourself behaving coolly, calmly and quietly ... look at that happy smile on your face ... notice how calm and quiet it sounds ... notice how calm and confident you feel ... and how great it feels to have that calm and happy feeling of being in control of your voice ... you can shout if you want to ... you can whisper if you want to ... but most of the time I expect you will choose a calm, comfortable, controlled level ... which will be perfect for you.

I'm wondering what it's like to be so calm and happy and in control now that your unconscious mind has taken responsibility? ... And I'm wondering what the best thing for you is about being in control of your voice? ... And I'm wondering exactly what your mum and dad have to say? ... Well I don't really know ... although perhaps I can guess ... but I *do know that each day you feel more and more calm and confident* in yourself ... each day you *feel happy and confident in every situation* ... each day *you feel proud of yourself and pleased with yourself* ... knowing that *you are a boy/girl with very special abilities and you are very much in calm, quiet control of your mind ... calm, quiet control of everything about you.*

And now I think it is time for you to come back to the room here with me ... your fingers feeling perfectly normal ... neither too light nor too heavy ... you are feeing more and more wide awake and alert and aware that you have achieved something very special inside today which will have an amazing effect on your life as I count from 1 to 10 ... coming back ... wide awake ... wide awake ... well done (Child's Name).

Tic Script Extracts

The following may be included in scripts as appropriate to the symptoms and age of an individual child.

Calm a premonitory urge

Some sufferers are aware of a 'premonitory urge' immediately prior to the onset of a tic, which lets them know it is about to happen. These localised sensations are variously described by sufferers as: a build up of tension similar to the need to sneeze or scratch an itch, a sense of discomfort with a strong urge to blink, to clear the throat, to shrug the shoulders. A couple of extracts follow and these short frameworks can be adapted to suit the specific tic to be reduced or eliminated.

The urge to blink

As soon as you notice the sensation/feeling/discomfort/in your eye you will say the word *'calm'* and a wonderful feeling of calm will spread all over your face and all over your body and *that old urge to blink will fade right away* … right now … that's right … at first, you will actually say the word *'calm'* out loud and as you say the word *'calm'* the feelings will subside/calm down/fade away/disappear and *you will feel completely relaxed* … very soon you will only need to say the word *'calm'* silently in your head and the feelings will fade right away … right now … and *there will be absolutely no urge to blink* … and as the days and the weeks and the months go by … you will find more and more that … just *as soon as you begin to notice that sensation … the urge will disappear automatically* … the sensation/feeling itself has become a trigger for the urge to *disappear completely … the urge will disappear completely.*

The urge to clear the throat

As soon as you notice the sensation/feeling/discomfort/in your throat you will say the word *'calm'* and a wonderful feeling of calm will spread all over your face and all over your throat … all the muscles in your mouth and throat will relax and *that old urge to clear the throat will relax away … relax right away …* right now … that's right … at first, you will actually say the word *'calm'* and as you say the word *'calm'* the feelings will relax right away … and *you will feel completely relaxed* … completely at ease … completely calm … very soon you will only need to say the word *'calm'* silently in your head and the feelings will relax away … right away … right now … and *there will be absolutely no urge to clear the throat* … and as the days and the weeks and the months go by … you will find more and more that … *just as soon as you begin to notice that sensation/*feeling … *the urge will disappear automatically* … the sensation itself has become a trigger for the urge to *disappear completely … the urge will disappear completely.*

Note that in the following scripts there is intentional repetition of certain sections of text deemed to be useful for all the situations described.

Coping with your own feelings of embarrassment or shame

You understand that tics can affect quite a lot of people at different times in their lives … *they can come and they can go … a tic is something that can pass* … sometimes as quickly as it came … just like an itch … it can come and *it can go* … just like a thought … it can come and it can drift away and while *you are patiently waiting for it to pass … you can understand that tics are not your fault* … just like a cold *is not your fault* … just as a rash *is not your fault* … so if it should happen now and then … you will *take it in your stride* … it *won't bother you at all … it won't disturb you at all* … in fact … in a very funny kind of way … the more you even tried to care about it … the more you would *take it in your stride … as of no importance to you at all* … and the less importance it has … *the more easily it can disappear* … and while you are patiently … calmly … waiting for that to happen the more you can *be proud of yourself* for being able to *take it all in your stride* … it's just a small part of life … that no longer bothers you at all. ☞ **In your pre-trance discussion, elicit from the child and the parents some of the qualities or abilities that the child is proud of and include them as follows.** ☞ And often now … if you are daydreaming … you will find that your mind drifts on to what your mum said earlier … remember, she said that she is so proud of you because you are so very kind/thoughtful/caring and that you are the best boy/the most special girl/in the entire world … and she told me that it's great to have a son/daughter who has such a good sense of humour/who is so creative/who is so talented/who is so interesting/who is so interested in the world.

Coping with explaining about vocal tics to others

Now I know that you can understand that vocal tics (that's the name of that sound that happens in your throat) can affect quite a lot of people at different times in their lives … *tics can come and they can go … a tic/throat sound is something that can easily pass* … sometimes as quickly as it came … just like an itch … it can come and *it can go* … just like a thought … it can come and it can drift away and while *you are patiently waiting for it to pass … you can understand that these sounds are not your fault* … just like a cold *is not your fault* … just like a rash *is not your fault* … so if it should happen now and then … you will *take it in your stride* … it *won't bother you at all … it won't disturb you at all* … in fact … in a very funny kind of way … the more you even tried to care about it the more you would *take it in your stride … as of no importance to you at all* … and the less importance it has … *the more easily it can disappear* … and while you are patiently … calmly … waiting for that to happen the more you can *be proud of yourself* for being able to *explain it to other people in a very matter-of-fact kind of way* … it's just a small part of life … *you can explain it like this quite easily and calmly* … it's called a vocal tic, which means it is a sound that happens involuntarily … that means it is not done on purpose … it happens to you sometimes and it is just as much of a surprise to you as it is to them … you do not do it on purpose … you can ask them … to *please ignore it* … you can explain that it is something that usually goes away as children get older … but it can happen to anybody … anytime.

And by the way … it can happen to people who are very intelligent … and … of course … I know that you are very intelligent indeed.

And while you are patiently waiting for it to pass … and while you are practising all the relaxing at home … in that special way … and you are learning to relax the sounds away … just as you have done so fantastically well today … you will remember that there are many important things in life and you will find you *focus more and more on those other more interesting things as the sounds become less and less important to you.*

Dealing with people's responses to unintentional rude gestures or swearing

You yourself understand very well that TS/Coprolalia is an illness and it is not your fault … it is not your fault … so if it should happen now and then … you will *take it in your stride* … you will cope very coolly and calmly. Now you and I know that *it is not your fault* and we *know that you are learning to take more control over the sounds and take more control over the gestures … and take more control over the swearing* but we also know that many people know very little about this condition … in fact … *you are much more knowledgeable than they are* … and sometimes *it's good to explain to people what it is* … so they know what to expect and it won't surprise them so much … now, because *you are so knowledgeable … you are able to explain easily* that sometimes there will be sounds or movements or even rude words and swearing that happen when you least expect them … and *the best thing for them to do is to ignore it … you can explain easily and calmly* that it is a type of illness … and you really don't mean to be rude or to upset them in any way … *you really have no intention to offend them* … so ask them please to understand that you are very sorry if it sounds rude or if it's irritating but really the best thing for them to do is to *just ignore it.*

And now you are becoming more and more confident in yourself … more and more sure of yourself … more and more comfortable and confident on the inside and the outside … you will find it easier to explain/apologise to anybody … it becomes easier to explain each time you do it, whether it is to someone you know or someone you don't know … whether they are older or younger than you.

Cope with other people's teasing or unkind comments

You may also include a full ego-strengthening script and suitable extracts from a script in Chapter 11 on bullying.

And now *you are becoming more and more confident in yourself each day* … more and more sure of yourself … more and more comfortable and confident on the inside and the outside … and because you are so much more knowledgeable than you used to be … you know that some people do not really understand about TS as well as you do … and because they don't understand it, they sometimes make unkind or hurtful comments … but *you are able to cope with that teasing/those comments in a strong and confident way … and you absolutely refuse to let it bother you in any way … in fact, if ever you hear that teasing … you automatically remind yourself … that they don't really know about it and they don't understand it … you know and understand it far better than they do … and sometimes you choose to explain about it … staying cool and calm … and sometimes you just choose to ignore the things those people say … just in the same way as you are learning to ignore the tics themselves.*

You are strong inside … you feel good about yourself inside … you can focus on something worthwhile … focus on something really interesting as if you hardly hear what they say … the words are of no importance to you at all … you will find it easier to explain about TS to anybody … easier to explain each time you do it … whether it is to someone you know or to someone you don't know … whether they are older or younger than you … each day you are getting so much more confident than you used to be … and you will notice this confidence spread into every area of your life.

Habits Script: Stop sucking your thumb

Age range: approximately 4–7/8 years

This script works well for a 'girlie' type of girl but it could be adapted to include wizards and princes to appeal more to boys.

Choose any suitable short, relaxing induction.

I'm going to tell you a story about the fairy family who live at the bottom of my garden. The fairy king and queen live there with their two little daughters, the fairy princesses, Sophia and Maria, who are both very pretty. One day Sophia was wearing a blue fairy skirt, which was very sparkly and had a matching sparkly pale blue top, which had some holes for her beautiful golden wings at the back. She had on her best sparkly tiara in her hair and was as pretty as a picture. On her feet were her very best delicate fairy shoes because Princess Sophia always likes to look her best wherever she is.

Princess Maria was there too and, as you know, she is also very pretty … but … look at her! Pink skirt, green top, blue socks and she's got/wearing her clumpy red trainers on her feet … and where is her tiara? … She's quite forgotten it today.

The thing about Princess Maria is that she is very forgetful. She forgets where she has left her fairy shoes. She forgets that she looks so pretty when all her clothes match and so she puts on any old clothes with colours that really don't go together. She's always thinking about other things. She even forgets to *stop her thumb from going into* her *mouth* … but she really *does* … *want to stop.*

And because she really does … *want to stop* … she asked her sister, who had managed to *stop sucking her thumb* quite a long time ago, to help her remember to *stop sucking her thumb too* … Princess Sophia told her to do the same as she does … to listen to a special voice inside that reminds her … 'remember to *stop sucking your thumb*' it says 'remember you *never suck your thumb any more*' … it says … 'you've *had quite enough of that old thumb sucking habit … it was all wet and slimy* … and *you just don't want that old habit any more*'.

'So little sister,' said Princess Sophia to Princess Maria, … 'you can do that too … and you can be happy too … just like me, knowing that you can … *stop that old thumb sucking habit … once and for all* … and if ever you even begin to feel your thumb lifting up to your mouth … you just … *listen to that inside voice* … and it will remind you that *your hands and your thumb feel so comfortable and dry … now* that you've managed to *stop sucking your thumb* … and then your thumb will come right back down into your lap … so little sister … *you need to listen to your own inside voice … and then there will be no more thumb sucking … I know you've had quite enough of that old habit* … if your thumb starts to go up to your mouth … your other hand will just *move over and help that hand down from your mouth* … and *your thumb will feel so comfy in your other hand* that you can *let it stay there … feeling all comfortable and calm and relaxed* … you will *be so happy that you have taken charge of your thumb* … you will *feel so grown up now and so proud of yourself*.'

Princess Maria thought it was a great idea but she was a little bit worried that she might forget about it so Princess Sophia thought and thought and thought about it and finally came up with the answer. That night when Princess Maria was in bed and *feeling very sleepy and dreamy* … Princess Sophia sprinkled some of her very special fairy dust on her and whispered the magic words … 'Sparkling Fairy Dust, to work your magic is a must' … and then in the morning Princess Maria's memory got *better and better … and each day* … she began to *remember to stop sucking her thumb* … and remember everything more easily … so now, if you see them both in the garden, it is difficult to know who is Maria and who is Sophia because neither of them has her thumb anywhere near her mouth … they both look so pretty and sparkly and Maria has remembered her tiara … and her clothes all match nicely and Maria's hands are … just as calm and comfortable as Sophia's now she has *remember*ed to … *stop sucking her thumb.*

So (Child's Name) when you go to bed tonight, I think both the fairy princesses will come to visit you when you are asleep … in fact, they could even do it now … and sprinkle their magic dust on you and whisper their magic words … 'Sparkling Fairy Dust, to work your magic is a must, (Child's Name) is grown up you know, so sucking thumbs has got to go' … and then you can have a wonderful dream of how brilliant things are for you … now *you have stopped sucking your thumb* … just like Princesses Sophia and Maria …. you can dream about how wonderfully happy you are now when you're watching television/in the car and both your hands are just holding your teddy/holding that toy/sitting in your lap … and you feel so calm and comfy and relaxed that you *forget about that old thumb altogether* … *you are so proud of yourself* that *you have stopped that old habit so easily* and of course mummy and daddy are so proud of you too … isn't it good that even when *you are tired and sleepy* … you *never think about that old thumb* any more because *you feel so relaxed and comfy* … you are so pleased that it isn't pushing your teeth out any more … and even when you're in bed at night … look at you … you're all cuddled up with teddy/your dolls/your animals and you *hardly ever think about it at all* except to think *how happy and proud you are.*

And of course since *you got really fed up with that boring, old habit* it doesn't matter if you are in a good mood or a bad mood … if you are wide awake or tired and sleepy … at home or at school … in the car or in bed or anywhere at all … it doesn't make any difference to you and your thumb at all … you are just so happy and pleased with yourself …and *how grown up you are* … and I wonder what nanny and granddad (as appropriate) are going to say? Look at nanny's face when she notices that there is something a bit different about you … did she notice it first all by herself or did you tell her to guess what *amazing thing you have managed to do all by yourself*?

Chapter Seven

Anxiety

The Nature of Anxiety

Anxiety is a state with three component parts: psychological, physical and behavioural.

Psychological

There are anxious thoughts, sometimes obsessive, focused on anticipated events, which may be real or imagined, and are often related to impending doom or disaster.

Physical

Symptoms may include shortness of breath, dizziness, increased heart rate, trembling, muscle tension, sweating, numbness, tingling, dry mouth, abdominal discomfort, nausea, fatigue, full-blown panic attack.

Behavioural

Symptoms may include crying, screaming, tantrums, avoidance behaviour, e.g., not going into or fleeing from a frightening situation, performing an overt or covert avoidance ritual, sleeping difficulties, refusal to be parted from a parent or caregiver, restlessness, irritability, compulsions and obsessions.

Origins of Anxiety

Genetics, Learning History, Biological Theory, Physical Causes, Emotional Distress

Some anxiety disorders have a tendency to run in families; this is very likely to be due in part to a genetic predisposition but it may also be partly due to the fact that we tend to model the behaviour of those around us. In other words, children who see their parents respond in a certain manner may tend to reproduce some similar behaviour. Risk of developing a panic disorder increases by 10–20% if there is an immediate relative suffering from the condition.

- Our environment, such as an early or ongoing domineering (or abusive) upbringing, may contribute to a generally over-anxious disposition. Conversely, caring, overprotective parents who are alert to any possible lurking danger can also contribute to anxious dispositions in their children.

- Very rarely there may be a physical cause, e.g., a tumour of the adrenal gland. Another example could be changes in the rhythm of the heart. Although this is more common in adults, it can, rarely, occur in children and can mimic a panic attack. These physical causes should be diagnosed, assessed and managed by a medical practitioner.

- Certain side effects of, or withdrawal from, prescription drugs (or even simple cold and flu remedies) can cause anxiety, as can 'recreational' drugs, including alcohol and caffeine.

- Life-altering events, such as death (even of a pet), divorce, disharmony in family or friendships, a new baby, moving, changing schools, single or repeated traumatic events, and natural disasters or frightening crimes repeatedly reported on television news, are frequent causes of anxiety in children.

- Several weeks or months of stress or illness may initiate panic attacks.

- The biological theory presupposes a chemical imbalance in the brain, which can be addressed through medication, preferably in conjunction with a talking therapy.

What Maintains Anxiety?

Association and Generalisation

Something relatively harmless can become associated with something unpleasant or scary, for example, a nurse's uniform can be associated with a fear of injections and so a child can become frightened of all nurses. This fear can then be further associated with other places, objects or people, and generalised out to the extreme extent that a child won't walk past a hospital because nurses work there.

Avoidance

If children continually avoid putting themselves into a situation that they perceive as frightening, they never give themselves a chance to find out that, in fact, they are able to cope with it and it isn't as bad as they feared. In this way the fear becomes more intense because the situation is now perceived as something so alarming that it is impossible even to attempt to deal with it.

Reinforcement

A fear may be reinforced through the very act of avoidance, for example, if a child is taken to school and is so frightened that he or she is brought home again without going inside, the ensuing feeling of relief they get reinforces the fear. Another form of reinforcement is through something called secondary gain, for instance, if a child who is frightened of the dark is continually allowed to spend the night in the parents' bed, the fear is rewarded and therefore strengthened. Even just too much attention and cuddling every time the child is a tiny bit apprehensive can reward and reinforce their apprehension.

Common Forms of Anxiety

Generalised Anxiety Disorder (GAD)

Children with GAD tend to worry about almost everything and have recurring fears and anxieties. They are often very eager to please and have perfectionist tendencies.

Separation Anxiety Disorder
(dealt with in more detail in Chapter 8)

Children with separation anxiety disorder display intense anxiety about being away from their caregivers or from their home.

Obsessive-Compulsive Disorder (OCD)
(dealt with in more detail in Chapter 9)

Children with OCD experience obsessions and compulsions that can begin in early childhood or adolescence. These cause a great deal of anxiety and can take up so much time that they interfere with daily living.

Social Phobia

Social phobia usually begins in teenage years although it is not uncommon to find it in younger children too. Children may have a constant fear of social situations and speaking in front of others and tend to avoid situations that involve social contact.

Post-Traumatic Stress Disorder (PTSD)

Children may develop PTSD after experiencing or witnessing physical or emotional trauma such as disaster, physical, emotional or sexual abuse, or being involved in an accident. They can also be traumatised by an event that can seem mild to an adult since children are not mature enough to understand the bigger picture.

Mild air turbulence during a flight or a parent being hospitalised, for example, may be terrifying because the child interprets these as leading to certain death. The trauma may be continually replayed through nightmares and imaginative play. These children will usually experience symptoms of general anxiety, particularly displaying the startle response, irritability, going off their food and being fearful of sleeping alone.

Panic Disorder

Children and adolescents with panic disorder suffer from frequent panic attacks that can last for just a few minutes or for several hours. Such attacks often begin during adolescence but are sometimes seen earlier. Children become so fearful of the fear itself that their life becomes severely restricted in terms of activities and in places they will visit.

Common Childhood Apprehensions

It is common for children to display mild anxiety about events that are new or challenging. These anxieties will normally respond very easily to hypnotherapy treatment. In severe or resistant cases, it is wise to refer for a psychological assessment.

Referral to a Medical Practitioner

If there is no obvious cause and the anxiety does not reduce fairly quickly with hypnotherapy, it is advisable to refer to a medical practitioner just to rule out the very rare cases, as mentioned earlier, of an underlying physical cause. Where there is, as expected, no organic cause, hypnotherapy can be very effective for reducing or eliminating fears and installing and maintaining new, calmer responses.

Suitable Aims for Hypnotherapy Treatment

- Dispel fears of dying or going mad. Explain the fight or flight response.
- Reframe anxiety as an overenthusiastic reaction by the inner mind designed to help protect them.
- Build confidence and self-esteem.
- Eliminate or reduce anxiety or phobia.
- Increase calm and relaxation.
- Encourage thought-stopping and positive self-talk.
- Deal with possible related problems such as OCD.

Suitable Interventions

- Use short inductions that take the focus away from the body and involve the imagination and visual element from the outset, interweaving indirect suggestions for calm and control early on. After the child shows signs of being absorbed in the process, you can introduce a relaxation deepener.

- Direct suggestions for calm and control.

- Any metaphor for letting go of worries.

- Any metaphor where children can get a sense of control and manipulate symptoms, such as 'master control room' or 'computer' (see Chapter 6, 'Spaceship master controls').

- Rewind procedures, used in or out of formal trance.

- Desensitisation and exposure.

- Delay the anxiety response. (Delaying the response gives a degree of control and makes it then easier to eliminate the response altogether.)

- Thought-stopping (see Chapter 9, 'Thought-stopping on your computer mind').

- Visualisation with sub-modality change (see Chapter 11, 'Shrink the Bully' and Chapter 10 on fear of monsters).

- Guided visualisation of successful handling of the problem.

- Anchors (triggers) for calm.

Teaching Coping Strategies

In addition to hypnotherapy treatment itself, it is useful to teach children one or more coping strategies that they can use should they feel the need. I tell them it is a bit like using a sticking plaster while the cut on their finger is healing. There is a selection of strategies in the next box that will appeal to different age groups and different personalities.

Breathing

People are often told that they need to breathe deeply and, while it is true that we should practise relaxed breathing from the abdomen rather than shallow breathing from the chest, this instruction is often misinterpreted by the child as a need to take in more oxygen. They then start to breathe in through their mouths, which will have the effect of encouraging hyperventilation and yet more panic – the very thing they are seeking to control! What they need to practise is *controlled breathing*.

If they are having a panic attack, they can use the 'cupped hands breathing technique' described in the next box, which may help to re-establish the very delicate balance of oxygen and carbon dioxide in the blood, and thereafter to the brain. It also gives them something to do which will both distract them and give them a sense of taking control.

> **Coping Strategies for Children**
>
> Select the strategy according to the maturity of the child and simplify when necessary for very young children.
>
> **Controlled breathing (for older children)**
> When people are shocked or frightened by something, the natural response can be to gasp. This gasp comes in the middle of your normal breathing cycle, NOT when you really need to breathe in. The truth is that you already have enough breath in your lungs and the reason that you think you can't breathe is because you are trying to

take in air when you already have more than enough. So, remember you may need to breathe OUT before you can breathe in!

When people keep breathing in through an open mouth they may hyperventilate (over breathe), which can in itself cause all the physical panicky feelings in their body. Sometimes people feel as if they are unable to 'catch their breath' or get tingling feelings, or even feelings of cramp, in the face, hands or feet. These panicky feelings can then make them feel they want to 'over breathe' even more than before. So, the really important thing to remember is to close your mouth and breathe through your nose to slow down and control your breathing.

Put your hand on your lower abdomen and feel it rising as you breathe in, just as if you were blowing up a balloon. If it doesn't rise, you are breathing from your chest. Count to 4 as you breathe in, always through the nose with your mouth closed, and count to 4 as you breathe out. Take five to ten controlled breaths in this way and you will find you gain good control of your feelings.

Ratio breathing

Close your mouth, and count to yourself as you breathe in to the count of 3 and out to the count of 6. Continue to do this until you feel more in control again.

Breathe in: 1, 2, 3, Breathe out: 1, 2, 3, 4, 5, 6.

Cupped hands breathing

If you feel really panicky, put your cupped hands over your nose and mouth and breathe in the air you have just breathed out. This can help to bring back up the levels of CO_2 towards normal and make you feel calmer. It is best to do it with your mouth closed and you can do it anywhere without people taking any notice of you.

Tapping your inner wrist in time to your heartbeat

If you get worried because you can feel your heart beating fast, first of all remember that it's good your heart is beating so well; the time to worry would be if it wasn't beating! Second, begin to tap your inner wrist in time with your heart beat and very soon you will find the heartbeat begins to slow back down to normal.

Count backwards

If you get worried because you can feel your heart beating fast, at the same time as breathing in through your nose with your mouth shut, start counting slowly backwards in your head from 200. (200, 199, 198, 197 ...) and notice which number you get to when your heartbeat begins to slow down.

Remember the number (you might want to write it down) so you notice if you ever do it again that you probably calm down more quickly than you did the last time.

Move about

Shake your hands and/or your feet quite violently/jump about/stretch up and then bend down/go for a walk. This releases adrenaline and makes you feel much better.

Distract yourself

Do a practical task, count backwards from 100 in 3s, talk to someone.

Keep a panic-diary and record where you are, what you were doing or thinking about before the feeling started and how long it takes for the feeling to calm down. Carry a notebook and pen with you to write down the information. This way, you not only give yourself something else to do, you also have some very useful information to tell your therapist.

Eat something

Eat something like an apple or a banana or piece of cheese. Avoid sugary snacks as they quickly send your blood sugar up and down, which can make you feel worse.

Identify your feelings and thoughts, and then challenge them (for use with older children whom you have already taught some ideas from Cognitive Behaviour Therapy).

Remember to ask yourself these questions:

- What feelings are you experiencing?
- What are the thoughts that triggered the feeling?

Challenge the thoughts in the same way as you have done with your therapist

- *Of course I'm not going to die! In fact these are the normal symptoms of the 'Fight or Flight Response' my therapist told me about. I must remember to use my coping strategy.*

- *So what if I faint? If I were to faint (not very likely,) what is the worst that could happen? People don't die of fainting; they just feel horrendous at the time. Someone would help me get up and if nobody did, I would wait and then get up on my own.*

- *So what if I was actually sick? (I never have really been sick.) Someone would help.*

- *So what if it's embarrassing? I can put up with a bit of embarrassment. Other people do different embarrassing things and most people feel sorry for them.*

- *It happened before and I was fine afterwards. I'll be fine this time too.*

Use a coping statement

- I know I can stay cool, calm and in control.

- I don't like this feeling but I know I can cope with it anyway.

- Although these feelings are a bit scary, they will soon pass.

- Everyday I am learning to cope better and better.

- Everyday I am getting stronger and stronger.

- I am not going crazy. This is panic talking … not me!

Use your calm triggers

Remember to use the calm triggers, for example, the finger and thumb gesture you learned during your hypnotherapy session (see page 110).

Anxiety Script: Rewind procedure

Age range: Any age, with suitable adaptation to language

There are many variations on this theme, which is based on dissociation and guided visualisation in a way that breaks up the original coding of the memory in the brain. We remember things in words, sounds, pictures, feelings, and sometimes smells and tastes too, and naturally we normally remember them in the sequence they occurred. If we play about with the sequencing, the colours, the size and any other variable that you can think of, the memory trace we store in our brains and any associated negative feelings are altered, in some cases quite dramatically. This is normally the first intervention I use for situations in which one or more specific frightening events have triggered anxiety or panic. The procedure can be carried out with or without formal trance.

NB If you choose to use this type of intervention with a traumatic or tragic incident, it would clearly be inappropriate to use some of the suggestions for modality change made in the middle of this script. Read it through thoroughly before use and select from the dissociation techniques that follow the script.

To check that the child understands the procedure, demonstrate it first on a memory that contains no upsetting content, such as the journey to see you, which will be clear in his or her mind.

Demonstration of technique

How did you come to see me today? ... Can you see that journey in your mind/in your imagination/on your mental television from the moment you left your house to the moment you arrived at my front door? Some people find they can see it better when they close their eyes ... you do it how you like ... just see it through and tell me when you see yourself arriving at my front door ... great. Tell me, did you see yourself as if you were watching an actor on the television? ... Good. You did that so well that you are going to find the next part very easy. Call up that picture of you and mummy at my front door ... and now I want you imagine that you are holding the remote control in your hand and when I count to 3, I want you to press the rewind button and watch everything happening backwards and quite quickly too ... just as it does when you press the rewind button while you're watching a DVD at home. I want you to watch it going all the way back till you get back to your own front door ... but remember this time you will be going backwards all the way home, you'll be walking backwards up the path and the car will be driving backwards all the way home ... Are you ready? 1, 2, 3, go! ... ... Great you're back home again. You did that brilliantly (Child's Name).

Rewind script to use for the problem

Now you know exactly how to do the thing we are going to do next ... so we can *change all the bad/scary/upsetting feelings* that you had when the fire happened/you went to school/Jane was sick/those boys were teasing you. Of course you will remember that it all happened but you will be able to *remember it in a way that is more comfortable and feels safe … remember it in a way that is calmer and easier.* Would you like that? … Okay. Let's do it. I want you to tell me what you were doing before it all happened when you were feeling perfectly safe/happy/Okay … Good. That's going to be the exact beginning of our movie/film/TV programme. But later I know things began to go wrong, didn't they? … But what I want you to tell me right now is exactly when you were *feeling perfectly safe/happy/Okay once again* … Good. So when you got back into the house/car/garden/wherever you were *feeling perfectly safe again … you are perfectly okay back in the house/car/garden … and that is going to be the end* of our movie/film.

Կ **At this point you could introduce more elements of dissociation if you want to. A selection of dissociation processes follows the script. As a rule of thumb, the more frightening the incident, the more dissociation you want to achieve. In cases of trauma, for example, you might want to introduce several safeguards to enable the child to feel able to go through the process without being re-traumatised.** Կ

Let's start by looking at the beginning of the film where you are safe and feeling fine. Got that picture? Good … now see the whole film through from beginning to end and tell me when you've got the picture of you at the end of the movie/film, feeling perfectly safe back in the house/car/garden/wherever … good … very well done indeed, (Child's Name).

Now blank out that screen for a moment or two before we begin to *change all those old unwanted feelings into more positive ones* … great … now get the very end safe picture up onto the screen once again and press the rewind switch and watch it all going backwards from the end to the beginning … quite quickly … just like when you rewind something at home … tell me when you are back at the beginning of the film where you *feel perfectly safe* playing with your toys/watching the TV. Well done.

Now we're going to do that again but we're going to make some other changes, because you've got some other buttons on your remote control that you didn't even know you had … are you ready? Can you see the safe end-picture? When I say *1, 2, 3, go* … you're going to press the rewind and also the colour-change button and … hey … that's amazing … everybody turns into different colours … there could be yellow faces with pink spots and green faces with red stripes … I want you to notice all the different colours and tell me afterwards what they were … are you ready? 1, 2, 3, go.

Well done. You're back playing with your toys/watching TV feeling perfectly safe … What colours were people's faces? What difference did that make? Oh, it didn't seem so scary … that's good, isn't it? Very well done.

106

♋

- Each time you run the movie on rewind, stress the aspect of 'feeling safe' at the beginning and end.

- Repeat the procedure at least four or five times, making more changes to modalities with each rewind.

- Change the size of the characters, making the child bigger or smaller as appropriate. Usually the bigger the size of the child and the smaller the size of any threatening people or objects, the more empowered the child will feel.

- Turn everybody into cartoon characters, with the child being his or her favourite character, of course.

- Introduce jolly music in the child's imagination (or in reality)/get him or her to imagine singing a favourite song/get the parent to sing along with you in a rendition of 'Happy Birthday to You'.

- Increase the speed of the rewind.

Optional insertion

- After having carried out the rewind procedure on screen (dissociated), you can ask the child to mentally step into the film and imagine actually being there (associated) carrying everything out backwards.

♋

Now I would like you to call up the picture of you at the beginning of the film, playing with your toys/watching TV … looking exactly like your normal self … no funny colours … no cartoons this time … and I want you to go through it forwards this time at normal speed from the beginning to the end and have yourself react coolly and calmly … just as you would have wanted to do … and when you get to the end and you are feeling absolutely fine … I want you to tell me what was different about it this time.

So this time it felt better/you felt calmer/you felt more in control/it even seemed funny! … Wonderful! … Could you improve it/make it better in any way? If so, just run it through in your mind making any improvements at all in the way you reacted … so you can keep this memory in your mind … which *is altogether easier for you*, is it not?

♋ **Be prepared to repeat this procedure several times until the child is satisfied that his or her behaviour in the movie can't be improved in any way. You can also get the child to run it through on fast forward several times to reinforce the new memory.** ♋

And … just before we finish … the very last thing I want you to do is to jump into the picture and be there now and go through the whole thing from beginning to end … noticing how differently you handle everything now … how you feel confident inside and in control of your feelings … brilliant … you are fantastic!

Summary of Rewind Procedure

1. Prepare to turn the frightening event into a film/movie and establish a safe beginning and a safe end.

2. See the film through on a mental television screen from beginning to end (Optional: create further dissociation by sitting above/beside self to watch whole process). Freeze-frame the safe end scene.

3. Run the film backwards as if on rewind mode, emphasising the safe end and safe beginning. Blank out the screen.

4. Repeat Rewind Procedure, changing modalities of speed, size, colour, cartoons, and so forth, blanking out the screen between each rewind.

5. Optional: step into the end scene of the film (associated) and rewind it again.

6. Run the film forwards again from the beginning, ensuring that the child behaves as he or she would prefer to have done (dissociated). Repeat this action until no further improvements can be made and the child reports that previous negative feelings have been eliminated or significantly reduced.

7. Have the child jump into the picture and go through the event from beginning to end, noticing the feelings of confidence and calm (associated).

Ideas to increase the process of dissociation

(These suggestions are particularly useful in cases of trauma. NB Always remember that you can ask the child directly to tell you how he or she will feel most protected while doing these tasks in his or her imagination.)

Ask child clients to:

- float off to a favourite, safe place.

- imagine they are sitting beside/behind/above themselves, watching themselves looking at a television/computer screen.

- put as many imaginary curtains or blinds in front of the television set as required to allow them to feel capable of watching the screen. They can then remove screens one at a time, as they feel more able. In the case of a tragic or abusive event, this could be done over several sessions.

- imagine it happening to a child with a featureless face or stick figure so it is less immediately recognizable as themselves.

- imagine the television set in another room.

- run the film without sound, or have a soundtrack without pictures as appropriate to the individual child.

- imagine putting on an imaginary suit of armour/invisible shield of protection before doing any of the above.

- imagine it happening with someone they trust at their side, possibly holding their hand (mum/dad/sibling/a grown-up self/a hero/you, the therapist) and helping them get through the situation safely, or as best they can under the circumstances.

Anchors

Anchors are essentially powerful triggers for a behavioural response, associated with something already experienced, and can be positive or negative; negative, as in the case of seeing a syringe, smelling the antiseptic and immediately feeling faint; positive as in the case of hearing a snatch of 'your song' and being put into a good mood because it transports you to a wonderful time from long ago. Anchors come in all kinds of shapes and sizes; something you see, hear, feel, smell or taste can cause an instant reaction.

In real life, anchors are accidental – they just happen and we respond to them naturally – but in hypnotherapy, we deliberately aim to take the power away from negative anchors that underlie many fears and phobias. Conversely, we aim to empower people by giving them positive anchors to trigger resourceful states. Sometimes empowerment may be in the form of simply reminding them of a time when they scored a goal or got a fantastic exam result in order to allow them to re-access that feeling in the moment. Other times, the process may involve a more structured approach in which they are given a gesture, which they can reproduce at will to trigger a resource state whenever they need it. The script 'Treasure hunt' makes use of anchors but you can use the procedure outlined in the next box with or without a formal trance state.

Setting an anchor

1. Decide which trigger you will use, perhaps squeezing the finger and thumb together, squeezing your fist or taking a deep breath. It needs to be something that can be remembered and reproduced exactly while also being unobtrusive so other people will not notice what is being done.

2. Decide which resource state is appropriate to be triggered, such as confidence/calm/enthusiasm.

3. Close your eyes and think of a time when you remember feeling particularly confident/calm. Let yourself remember exactly what that felt like and experience it all over again in your mind. Bring back the feelings, remember what you could see around you and see that picture in your mind again, maybe remembering what

you were hearing at the time, and fully imagine it happening to you right now. As the memory and the experience get stronger, set the chosen trigger, for example, squeeze your finger and thumb together, and capture the feeling in your fingers as you link it with the remembered experience. You can also see the same picture in your mind's eye and say a word or phrase to yourself at the same time – Calm/Stay cool/Go for it!

4. Open your eyes and let the gesture go before the positive feeling begins to fade. You want to keep the link as strong as you can.

5. Repeat Steps 3 and 4 three times.

6. Test the anchor. Make the gesture or take a deep breath, say the word or phrase to yourself, see that picture in your mind and notice how it brings back that positive feeling. If it fails to do so or isn't strong enough, repeat Steps 3 and 4 until it works.

7. Once you have tested it and found it works, you can rehearse using the anchor in the situation in which you want to feel confident or calm or whichever resourceful state is desired. Do a guided visualisation and practise firing the anchor as many times as you can so it strengthens the anchor for use in the real world whenever it is required.

8. Use the anchor often; frequent use will strengthen not weaken it.

Anxiety Script: Throw anxious feelings into the bin

Age range: approximately 4–8 years

This script uses the idea of a 'soft play centre' so check with the parents regarding whether or not their child is familiar with these centres before you choose to use it. When using the script, remember that most children will probably know such a centre by the particular name of the one they visit, so ask the parents beforehand for that name.

Let's do some imagining (Child's Name) … Look at the wall over there and tell me when you can imagine lots of soft, brightly coloured bouncy balls … good … what colour are they? … Right … so you can keep looking at those or … if you'd like to … you can *let your eyes close* because with your eyes closed *it is even easier to imagine things,* don't you think? … You could imagine you are in one of those soft play centres where all the sides are made of strong net which *keeps you very safe* ... but they're very soft if you fall against them and you can just bounce back and land on hundreds of really soft, squashy, brightly coloured balls ... one of those places where there are little slides to slide down ... and cubes/boxes with big holes in the sides to climb through ... nod your head when you can imagine you're there now ... great.

This place is a very special place because it's a place where you go when you want to (Child's Name) *leave any nervous feelings or scary thoughts* behind you ... you can leave all those scared feelings you told me about and *come out with strong, brave feelings instead* ... and you can *do that now* ... the first place to go is over to those little steps ... climb up the steps and you'll find a big yellow bin ... this is where you throw all the feelings you really don't want any more ... so first of all you have to remember exactly what they are ... that's right, those are the ones ... the ones you *used to* feel when you went into school/went to your friend's house/went to a party ... not nice, are they? ... You don't want those old feelings any more, do you? ... Are you ready to throw them away? ... Good ... you can tip them into the bin ... can you hear them clattering/whooshing all the way down to the bottom? ... Wonderful ... are there any more? ... Have a look in your pockets to make sure you get them all ... and once you've thrown them all away ... just nod your head ... fantastic (Child's Name) ... you've done very well indeed.

Now you can walk over to the top of the slide ... sit down ... and slide all the way down ... feeling so free ... feeling so happy ... and when you get to the bottom ... you land on some more soft, squashy balls ... what colour are they? ... Pick yourself up and can you see that great big box over there with big holes in the sides? ... This is the box full of brave/confident/calm feelings ... as soon as you climb into it you are filled with these wonderful feelings ... what does that feel like? Is it amazing? ... Look over there ... there are some extra-strong brave feelings ... grab them and fill up all your pockets so you've got some extra-strong, brave ones ... now you can feel just how you want to *feel calm/relaxed and confident/brave and happy* (Child's Name) *all over and all the way through.*

So the next place to go is to that big red 'tomorrow/next week cube' over there with another big hole in it ... it's called a 'tomorrow/next week cube' because when you *step through the hole*, you will find you have climbed into tomorrow/next week with all the happy feelings you want inside you ... if you haven't already climbed inside ... do that now ... that's right ... you are walking into the classroom/going to your friend's house/going to the party feeling happy and confident/strong ... you've got all your brave feelings inside ... look at you! A big smile on your face ... you are chatting away to the other children ... what are you talking about? ☜ **Elaborate in lots more detail as appropriate to the relevant situations with the desired calm and confident feelings to reinforce the new behaviour.** ☜ You feel just as happy/brave/safe when you go to school/go to a party/go to your friend's house ... as when you're at home with mummy/daddy/teddy because now *you have thrown away all those* *old shy feelings you used to* have and filled yourself up with these wonderful feelings that let *you really enjoy yourself* … let you *really enjoy being you* … such a special boy/girl (Child's Name) … mummy and daddy think *you are amazingly special* … and I think you are very special too … and as you (open your eyes) feel your arms and legs wanting to wriggle around and have a very good stretch … perhaps you could tell me who else knows that *you are a very special person indeed*?

Anxiety Script: Lucky dip

Age range: approximately 5–8 years

Before use, elicit any previous positive experiences of fairs or visits to Disneyland in reality or on television, and revivify those memories. (Clearly, if a child has had negative previous experiences in this type of environment, this would not be an appropriate script to use.) To adapt the script for older children, you could keep the same basic concept but use the idea of a 'Bring and Buy' stall, or a 'New Feelings for Old' shop instead of a Lucky Dip stall if preferred.

Remember we were talking about fun fairs/Disneyland? I wonder if you can just *close your eyes and be there now in your mind.* … Have a walk around and see all the brightly coloured stalls/shops and Disney characters … is that Mickey Mouse/Snow White/Winnie the Pooh over there? … Look at all those rides … can you hear the sounds of people talking and laughing? … And the music … can you hear that too?

(Child's Name), look over there … there's a Lucky Dip stall with a very friendly looking Cinderella/Tigger/teddy bear selling tickets … do you know what a Lucky Dip is? … You buy a ticket and then you dip your hand inside a bucket/box/barrel/bag/and find a lucky present … you don't know what the present is till you pull it out. They've got some big, shiny, silver buckets with some very special 'feeling presents' inside … there are happy feelings and brave feelings and strong feelings and confident feelings and relaxed feelings … I wonder which of those you would like to have the most? … And, by the way … there's something very special about how you pay for your ticket … you don't use money … you use worries or scary feelings or problems instead … Cinderella/Tigger/teddy bear buys those old feelings you don't want and you get a Lucky Dip ticket instead … nod your head when you're ready to buy your ticket … great (Child's Name) … can you find all those old scary feelings? Get every last little one … look in your pockets … look in your tummy … look in your chest and in your throat … are there any hiding anywhere else? … In your head, perhaps? … Or in your legs? ☺ **Be sure to include the places where the child has already told you he or she experiences the frightened feelings.** ☺ Wonderful … that's good … Cinderella/Tigger/teddy bear wants them all before she/he gives you your ticket and she/he won't give them back, you know … be very sure you don't want them back … well done! Hand them all over then … nod your head when you've given every last little one away … now just check … all over your body and inside your mind … that *they are all gone* … wonderful … I guess that *feels so much better inside* now you've given them away … hold your hand out for your ticket … that's good.

So now it's time to put your hand inside and find your present … I wonder what feelings you're going to find … put your hand inside and fish around for the best bag of feelings you can find … and when you've got it … pull it out and let's read what it says on the bag … hey (Child's Name) that's amazing! You're really lucky … you must have paid a lot of scary feelings for that … you've won the very best present of all … you've got the bag of mixed feelings which means you've got some of all the good feelings there are in the whole wide world … you really did have a lucky dip, didn't you? You've got the whole lot! … You've got happy feelings and brave feelings and strong feelings and confident feelings and relaxed feelings … I wonder which of these you like best? … Put them into your pockets … breathe some of them inside you … put some into your tummy … put them wherever you need them … put them wherever they feel best … you are so, so lucky (Child's Name) … from now on whenever you go to school/go to bed/hear the thunder you will feel happy and feel brave and strong … and you will feel just as calm and relaxed as you are right now … just as I say you will … every day/night you will be remembering to use your 'lucky dip feelings' … and feel absolutely fine.

Just see yourself now in your mind … looking so fantastically happy and feeling so relaxed and calm. ☟ **Get the child to visualise feeling happy, brave and strong in the situations which he/she previously found frightening.** ☟ Now look at mummy/daddy/your teacher looking so surprised and proud of you … what are they saying? Yes that's right … they are so proud of you and they love you very much indeed and they are so glad you bought all those wonderful 'lucky dip feelings' that have made you such a happy little boy/girl.

And as you (open your eyes) feel your arms and legs wanting to wriggle around and have a very good stretch … perhaps you could tell me who else is going to know that *you are a very special ' lucky dip person' with ' lucky dip feelings' inside*?

Anxiety Script: Treasure hunt

Age range: approximately 8–12 years

When you use this particular induction you need to be sure you have cushions in the chair since it refers to receiving confidence through touching the cushions. If there are no cushions, you can substitute another induction and move directly to the second paragraph. The script uses finger and thumb anchors for calm and confidence within the framework of a treasure hunt. It works best if you elicit individual interests and strengths in your pre-induction talk so you can make use of these as treasure.

You can choose (Child's Name) whether you want to keep your eyes open as you *relax and listen to my voice* or whether you want to *let them close* so you can *listen* more comfortably and as you *let them close* you will probably *find that a rather nice sleepy feeling seems to start in your eyelids* and I don't know whether that is before or after you begin to *notice a rather nice feeling of snuggling down into the chair* … feeling the cushions underneath you … holding you up/propping you up/supporting you … and as you *sink down into those cushions* can you notice how that feels against your arms and legs … all soft and squashy … soft and squashy and silky/smooth/velvety/furry as you touch them with your fingers … and as you touch them with your fingers … can you *feel the sensation of the calm and confidence* already beginning to pass into your fingertips … spread into your fingers and up into your arms … and up into your shoulders … and up into your neck and head … and then down again … right down into your chest … down into your tummy … all the way down into your legs … and your feet … so nice to relax and feel the cushions holding you up/supporting you/propping you up like cushions full of calm and confidence … confidence … all around you … spreading into you … this is a nice way to *let calm and confident feelings replace those unwanted feelings* you told me about, don't you think … sinking deeper and deeper into the cushions and down into the chair … *more and more comfortable* with each word I speak … and as you *become more and more comfortable* … it *becomes easier to drift and dream.*

And drifting and dreaming … you can *drift off to* … a rather special park … with green, green grass and bright blue sky … where *today is a very special day* … there is going to be a treasure hunt … are you ready? … Look for the flag that says 'Treasure Hunt' and just underneath it, there are some instructions … take the winding path over there (to your right) and keep walking … until you notice there is a big tree with a small hollow in it … just about at your shoulder height … stand on your toes and put your hand inside and you will find a beautiful stone … your first piece of treasure! ☞ **All of this is normally done purely imaginatively, but with younger children it is also possible to have a small basket or bag to put their hand inside and find a nice polished stone as their treasure (a trigger/anchor) to take home. If you choose to do this, be aware that a real stone is easier to lose than an imaginative one!** ☜ This is a very special stone because … as you hold it now … really squeeze it … that's right … you can *notice a wonderful feeling of relaxation and calm* … can you feel it now? … Mmm, wonderful … and *every time you hold this stone in your hand and you give it a really good squeeze you will feel completely calm and relaxed* … this is your relaxing stone … wonderful … you are doing this so well … and every time you hear me say the word 'RELAX' I want you to squeeze that stone and *double the feeling of relaxation all over* … all the way through … so ready now … RELAX … wonderful.

And feeling incredibly relaxed right now … it's time to continue on your treasure hunt … the next instruction is to keep walking till you see a bridge over a little stream … let me know/nod your head when you get there … good … now walk over the bridge … can you see the baby ducklings in the water? … As you get to the other side … can you see the golden palace shining and glinting in the sunlight? … Look, there's a sign on the palace gate … it says 'No anxious feelings are allowed inside this palace … when you open the gate … you automatically *leave all anxious feelings outside'* … so … are you ready to go through? … Nod your head when you're ready … brilliant … and as you walk through … just notice how you *feel lighter and lighter* so you are almost floating through the gate … mmm … *squeeze your stone* … RELAX … doesn't that *feel wonderful?* … Floating up the steps and right into the entrance hall now … you're going to see a door … what does it say? Oh yes … (Child's Name)'s Treasure … this is the room that's got a special treasure chest of *all the confident feelings you'll ever need* … are you ready to open it up? … Open the lid and inside you'll find some golden pots of very special feelings.

☙ **This is where you use the child's own positive resources that you have elicited in your pre-induction talk. You can have pots full of the confident feelings experienced on the football field/when playing a musical instrument/writing a story/dancing/playing with a toy/playing on the PlayStation. You can have one pot or several pots; the child can borrow pots of confident feelings from a friend; you can give him or her a pot of confidence from a hero or from you. Provide as many as you think appropriate, and get the child to take a pinch and squeeze the feeling in between the finger and thumb each time. In this way, you are installing and reinforcing an anchor that he or she can use to trigger confidence when required.** ☙ Look, there's a lovely pot in the corner … this one contains all the amazing feelings you get when you play your saxophone/guitar/piano … open it up and take some of it in between your finger and thumb … just *capture all the feelings there right now … squeeze hard … just be there* … playing the music in your mind … be there now … hear the music … see what you see around you and *feel that wonderful feeling spreading all over you … you are so confident … see the amazing colour of confidence* and *keep it all in your finger and thumb right now* so that whenever you want an extra bit of confidence all you have to do is to … *squeeze your finger and thumb just like this* … and you will *feel all that confidence all over again* … just as strongly … just as powerfully … as *you are feeling so confident right now.* ☙ **Repeat with other resources as often as you think necessary.** ☙

Now it's time to leave through the exit at the back of the palace that leads on to the path of the future … and as soon as you actually *step onto the path of the future* … you will find it turns into the path of now … that's it … *step onto the path* … that's right … it has become the path of now … where *you have all the relaxed calm feelings you need* … you *have all the strong confident feelings you need* … just start by squeezing your stone/your fist with your special relaxing stone inside … RELAX … and *notice how calm and relaxed you feel.* ☙ **This is where you begin a guided visualisation of the child firing the finger and thumb anchors in situations he or she has previously identified as ones in which he or she would like to be calmer and more confident.** ☙

116

And because you told me you wanted some extra calm and confidence on the train/on the bus/in the car/etc. … just turn around and you will see that there is a small turning that leads to the station/the bus stop/the place where the car is parked etc. … and as you get onto the train/bus/into the car/etc. … you squeeze your finger and thumb together and *all those amazing confident feelings fill you up* … they fill you up so much that they overflow … you are surrounded with feelings of calm and confidence that *stay with you all through the journey* … and whenever you feel you want to have a little bit more confidence still … you just squeeze your finger and thumb together … and really *enjoy those feelings all over and all the way through* … and if ever you want to … RELAX a little bit more … you just squeeze your special stone … and you *feel just wonderful* … so as you continue your journey now … maybe looking out of the window … or reading a book … or chatting with your friends … do that squeezing if you want to … so you *enjoy going through the whole journey from beginning to end feeling absolutely fantastic.*

Now, I don't know whether you will tell anybody else about the special treasure that you found and what it has helped you to do … or whether it will be your secret … but I *do know* that you will *feel proud* that you have found your own very special way to *enjoy your journeys … happy … calm … relaxed … and very confident too …* and now I know that's it's time for you to come back from this particular journey … and come all the way back to the room with me as I count from 1 to 10 … feeling all the energy coming back into your body as I count … each number increasing your confidence … increasing your positive feelings about you.

Anxiety Script: Worry castles in the sand

Age range: approximately 8–12 years

Use a short 'Making yourself comfortable' induction.

I wonder just how quickly you (Child's Name) can allow yourself to *drift off in your imagination to a beach* … where it's sunny and warm … and if you *really think about it* you can probably *feel the sun on your skin* … and *notice the feeling of your feet on the sand* … and maybe as you look out at the sea you can just *hear the lapping of the water* as it comes in and up the shore and then … gently flows out again … the white bubbles of surf disappearing each time they flow back out again … from time to time perhaps you're feeling the cool water covering your toes … the blue sky is making the sea such a wonderful colour … and as you look up the beach … have you yet noticed those people building sandcastles not far from the water's edge? … Can you hear one of the boys asking, 'Why are you building the castles so near the water? Can't you see the water is going to wash them all away?' … 'But that's the whole idea,' one of them says … 'Don't you know about the worry castles? … You have to choose a spot … when the tide is coming in … far enough away for you to build your worry castle but near enough for you to know that quite soon the waves will

117

come in and smash all the castles down while you watch ... the water crumbles them all away ... the waves will keep coming in and out until all the worries are just soggy grains of sand and they all get washed away ... you *know it will happen* ... so you have to *be very sure* you want to *let all those anxious feelings go* ... because the sea ... *will ... take them all away*.'

Listen ...(Child's Name) they're all cheering as someone's worry castle is completely smashed away by a wave ... and the boy/girl ☞ **Choose the same sex as your patient.** ☜ is running happily off up the beach ... he/she's picking something up but I can't quite see what it is ... he/she looks very interested though ... he/she's putting it to his/her ear.

So maybe this will be a good place for *you to* (Child's Name) *let all those old scary/worried/frightened/anxious feelings go.* ☞ **You can refer directly to the child's fears.** ☜ Why not walk up the beach and find just the right spot for you to build your castle? ... You can make it a simple one or a very grand one ... it really doesn't matter ... you simply need to be sure that ... as you build it ... you dig out all those unwanted/jittery/fluttery/sick/anxious feelings inside of you ... all those unwanted thoughts ... and build them into your castle ... that's right ... pat them down firmly and *notice how it already feels better inside you ... lighter inside you ... now you have got them out of you* and into the sand ... some people even write any old thoughts that used to worry them in the sand too ... maybe you could do that too ... you can find an old stick somewhere that you can use ... and when *you have got all the old thoughts and feelings right out of you* ... you can stand back and wait for the waves to come in and wash them away ... maybe they'll do it with lots of little waves gently crumbling them away or perhaps there will be one of those spectacular ones that sometimes comes crashing in ... I don't know how *it will happen* ... but you can *certainly enjoy watching them all disappearing* into the sea.

And when *all those feelings have gone* ... when *those old fears are just a memory* ... nod your head ... because then it will be time to walk on up the beach following in the footsteps of the other children ... what are they looking for? ... Ah ... they're picking up shells and putting them to their ears ... one of the children is explaining something to the others ... listen ... 'Some of these are very, very old shells ... they have the wisdom of years and years and years in them' ... and when you need some help or some really good advice on how to (Child's Name) *cope better with things in your life* they give you the answer ... sometimes *you understand immediately what they say* ... and sometimes it's your inner mind that understands and *puts all the solutions in place while you sleep tonight* so that in the morning ... automatically you *know just what to do* ... you *know automatically just how to think and how to feel more calm ... more relaxed ... and more confident than ever before.*

So why don't you look for just the right shell? ... Nod your head when you've got it ... pick it up and hold it to your ear ... and listen hard for what it has to tell you ... your inner mind is listening too ... it's understanding everything ...

it's taking it all inside ... all the very wise words that will help you *take things completely in your stride from now on.*

And when you're ready ... you can take the shell with you, if you like ... so you can *listen again whenever you need to* ... and have you seen that little rock pool over there where the water is crystal clear? ... Walk over and have a look into the water ... look at your reflection ... now you can *see clearly (Child's Name) the change in you* ... clearly your inner mind was *listening very hard* because ... look at you ... *so cool and calm ... so confident and positive* ... look at how you are standing up so straight and so tall ... *your body is so relaxed, easy and comfortable* ... notice that big smile on your face that let's other people know too *how happy and confident you are inside.* ☜ **Now, use a guided visualisation of the child handling calmly the situations previously identified as those in which he or she wants to feel calmer and confident. Include other significant people such as family/friends/teachers showing positive reactions to his or her new behaviour.** ☞

Fantastic (Child's Name) ... you've done this so well ... perhaps ... now *you know how to do this so well* ... as well as going back to the beach in your mind and doing it for yourself if ever you want to ... you could be one of the helpful children who shows other people how they *can get rid of any worries if ever they need to* ... well done.

And now I think it's time for you to come back from your beach and find out how much easier it is to live your life feeling strong ... feeling relaxed ... feeling happy ... able to cope calmly and confidently with all the situations you face in your everyday life ... happier and more wide awake with each number as I count from 1 to 10.

Anxiety Script: Virtual reality

Age range: approximately 10 years upward

This script makes use of Ratio Breathing, the simple technique where you breathe in to the count of 3 and out to the count of 6, or in to the count of 4 and out to the count of 8. This can be taught in or out of trance as a coping mechanism to control anxious feelings. It is useful to set this as a homework activity to practise on a daily basis.

(Child's Name) settle yourself comfortably in the chair and let your eyes close and begin to imagine that the air around you is a wonderful colour of calm and comfort ... I wonder what colour that would be ... and as I count from 1 to 3 I'd like you to breathe in that wonderful calming, comforting colour so it spreads through your whole body ... are you ready? ... In 2, 3 ... Out 2, 3, 4, 5, 6 ... In 2, 3 ... Out 2, 3, 4, 5, 6 ... and each time you breathe out, you can breathe out any tension in your body ... breathe out any tension in your mind ... that's right .... breathing in 2, 3 ... Out 2, 3, 4, 5, 6 ... In 2, 3 ... Out 2, 3, 4, 5, 6 ...

and each time you do this ... your level of calm and comfort increases ... you become more and more relaxed ... you become more and more in control of your relaxation ... and this will continue as we go on.

So (Child's Name) I'd like you to notice that in front of you is a special (imaginary) virtual-reality helmet that I'd like you to put on ... that's right ... and now you are surrounded by a wonderful light and in front of you is a golden door that will only open into a healing garden when you *breathe calmly and deeply* and it senses *you are very calm and relaxed* ... let's try and see if it opens ... In 2, 3 ... Out 2, 3, 4, 5, 6 ... that's it ... nod your head when it opens. ☜ **If the child doesn't nod, do more calming breathing until he or she reports that the door opens. (In a worst-case scenario, you could improvise and let the child in by a side door but in practice I have never had anybody say it wouldn't open.)** ☞

That's brilliant ... well done ... now walk along the golden path till you reach a clearing where there is a man trying to light a bonfire ... the man is so pleased to see you because he needs your help ... this is a very unusual bonfire indeed ... it needs anxious/unhappy/unwanted/negative feelings to make it catch fire ... and this bonfire just needs some extra feelings to set it alight ... take a moment or two now to rest here for a while ... take a look inside yourself and find any negative/unwanted/anxious thoughts and feelings ... maybe you notice what colour they are ... what shape they are ... and begin to breathe them out of yourself and right onto the bonfire ... and when you (Child's Name) have breathed them all out onto the bonfire ... they will light the fire and *burn all those unwanted feelings right away* ... fantastic ... keep breathing and when you notice the fire catching light ... and then burning brightly ... you will know that *you have breathed all those negative feelings away* and when you *notice a light feeling inside as if a heavy weight has been lifted right off of you* ... it will be time for you to begin to stroll up the path again ... nod your head when you start walking up the golden path once more ... keep walking till you notice there is an enormous boulder blocking the path.

I believe you may need a bit of extra strength to move the boulder ... so ... luckily for you ... just to your left ... there is the well of strength ... with all the strong, confident feelings you need ... let that bucket down ... turning the handle round and round ... right down into the well ... further and further down to the very bottom... *you're probably sensing a bit of excitement now* ... and as you *fill up* your bucket *with all the strong, positive feelings* you need to help you *deal with all the situations you face in your daily life so much more easily than before* ... *so much more calmly than before* ... you can *feel excited* about what you will discover about yourself ... and as you wind the handle back the other way ... can you *notice how* ... already ... *you are feeling stronger?* ... Brilliant (Child's Name) ... the more you turn the handle, *the stronger you feel* ... *stronger and stronger* ... and when you have brought the bucket up ... take a drink and *know that you are strong enough to cope with anything that happens now* ... you may not *like every situation* that you meet but the amazing thing is that … from now on … you *notice yourself noticing how brilliantly you can deal with things now.*

Now, walk up to the big boulder/rock … and you will find it will move aside when *your mind is very calm and relaxed* … and you *feel strong and confident* … say the words to yourself now … calm and relaxed … I am calm and relaxed … I am strong and confident … now look at the boulder/rock and when *you are very calm indeed* … and when you *get a real sense of the feelings of internal strength and confidence* … it will gently move aside … say those words in your head again … I (Child's Name) am calm and relaxed …. I (Child's Name) am strong and confident … and nod your head when the boulder gently moves aside. ☋ **If the child doesn't nod, do more calming breathing or a suitable quick deepener, e.g., 10 to 1 deepener, till he or she reports that the boulder moves aside. (In a worst-case scenario, you could improvise and call in a strong, calm helper to assist with moving it to one side but, in practice, I have never had a child report that it refused to move.)** ☋

And now walking along the path you find it so natural to *be aware of feelings of calm and confidence* that … even in those situations which used to cause concern … *you are now able to manage them calmly … manage them confidently* … as you walk along you get a very real sense of being there in those situations you told me about … *behaving calmly … completely in control … your mind focusing on other things* which are far more interesting … your mind drifting on to the football match where you scored that amazing goal/your music/your plans for the weekend, etc. … If ever you want any extra calm and control … you *remember your ratio breathing* and gently, naturally finding yourself breathing … In 2, 3 … Out 2, 3, 4, 5, 6. ☋ **Include detailed guided visualisations of particular situations that have previously been identified by the child as ones in which he or she wants to feel calmer and more confident.** ☋

Well done (Child's Name) … you are now able to *cope calmly and confidently with all the situations you face in your everyday life* … and as I count from 1 to 10 and you *feel happier and more wide awake with each number* … the realisation becomes stronger and stronger that you can *truly enjoy your life so much more* now that you have left those old feelings in the past where they really belong.

Hypno-desensitisation

Hypno-desensitisation is an excellent technique for specific fears and phobias commonly used to great effect with adults. (This technique is clearly and fully explained by Ursula James in her *Clinical Hypnosis Textbook*). The technique is appreciated by 14- and 15-year-old clients, especially when they are told that this is something you usually do with adults but you feel that they are sufficiently mature to benefit from it. I find it is best to simplify and shorten the method, particularly when children are less than 14 years old, since most will not have the patience to go through as many detailed, graded scenarios as you might present to adults. In the development of a hierarchy of fearful situations (subjective units of disturbance scale [SUDS]), I would probably expect them to choose a maximum of five situations and with younger children it is useful to present a visual such as a ladder or a mountain and get them to indicate where their anxieties lie. I find young children are more likely to give a range of different situations with less precise understanding of hierarchical difference. In the case of older children I might make use of an ideomotor response (IMR), but with younger ones I would be content to ask them for a conscious head nod or finger lift to indicate their level of calm and comfort.

Procedure

1. Establish a modified SUD scale as in Figure 1.

2. Establish new, desired response.

3. Use any induction and deepener suitable to age.

4. Give direct suggestions for calm, safety and confidence as appropriate.

5. Present elicited scenarios of the child handling the situation as desired.

6. Get head nod, finger lift or ask the child to tell you when he or she feels comfortable and confident enough to move up the hierarchy to the next scene.

7. Repeat deepening and direct suggestions if necessary.

8. Continue presenting scenarios to the top of scale or to the point where the child is comfortable. If necessary, the scale can be resumed in a subsequent session.

9. Ego strengthening.

10. Wake up.

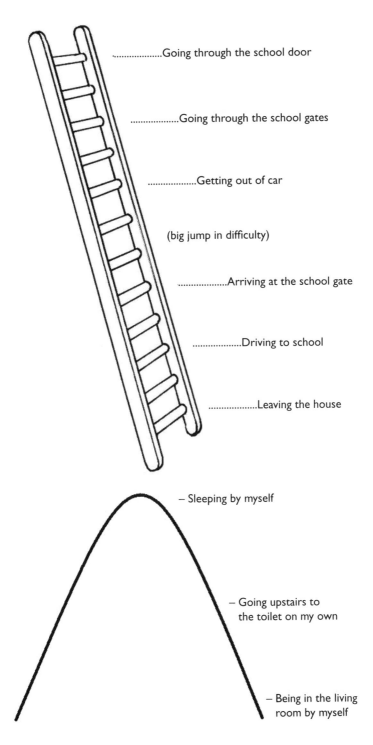

..................Going through the school door

..................Going through the school gates

..................Getting out of car

(big jump in difficulty)

..................Arriving at the school gate

..................Driving to school

..................Leaving the house

– Sleeping by myself

– Going upstairs to
the toilet on my own

– Being in the living
room by myself

Figure 1. Visual hierarchy of fears.

Chapter Eight

Separation Anxiety

Definitions, Signs and Symptoms

Separation anxiety refers to the distress that children experience when they are separated from their primary caregiver, usually the mother or father. Most children will suffer a degree of separation anxiety at some time in their early childhood as a natural part of development. It is only after it has become a serious problem that you are likely to see children present in your consulting room. At this level, it is possible that what is being experienced might be classified as Separation Anxiety Disorder, which is said to affect between 2% and 5% of children at any one time. This category includes anxiety that may have persisted for many months, or even years, or be experienced very intensely. In severe cases, children find being apart from a parent, even for a few minutes, intolerable and so will follow the parent from room to room. Bedtime can be a nightmare for all concerned as the child refuses to be left alone in his or her bedroom even when the parents are downstairs.

Although separation anxiety may become evident as early as age 6 months as a normal part of development, this chapter is focused only on cases that occur from 5 years old and upward. It may be that children have not grown out of earlier separation anxiety or that there has been a sudden onset of symptoms. Onset can occur at any time but most commonly appears between the ages of 7 and 9. Generally speaking, when children are accustomed early on to their parents working outside the home there seem to be fewer problems with this type of anxiety as they get older, although this is not always the case. By the age of 5 years old, the majority of children are able to leave their parents without significant distress for limited periods of time.

Referral to a medical practitioner

If there is no early improvement, referral to a medical practitioner should be advised in order to ensure that the problems are not symptoms of a condition that needs further physical or psychological investigation. As always, do not lead the parents to believe that you can totally cure the problem; rather, speak in terms of managing and lessening the severity of the symptoms and building confidence and self-esteem.

Possible Signs of Separation Anxiety Disorder

- Extreme anxiety or misery at being separated from parents or main caregivers.

- Excessive fear of parents being lost, kidnapped, hurt or even killed.

- Avoidance of going anywhere outside the home or away from parents (though there may be a limited number of people with whom they will stay, for example, grandparents with whom they have frequent and regular contact).

- Extreme anxiety even at the thought of parents leaving the house without them.

- Extreme anxiety at being left at home even though 'babysitters' are familiar and trusted.

- Extreme anxiety at being left at school.

- Extreme anxiety if parents should be late collecting them.

- Reluctance (or refusal in severe cases) to go to school.

- Reluctance or refusal to go to friends' houses, parties or sleepovers.

- Reluctance to attend clubs or sports activities on their own.

- Following a parent around at home.

- Demanding a parent stays with them at bedtime till they go to sleep.

- Demanding to sleep in the same room or bed with parents or appearing in their bedroom during the night.

- Nightmares, often about being lost and separated from parents, or about parents or the children themselves being hurt in accidents, crashes or fires.

Symptoms of the anxiety

- Crying
- Tummy aches
- Tantrums
- Sickness
- Headaches
- Diarrhoea
- Low self-esteem
- Breathing difficulty
- Panic attack with all its associated symptoms

Children vary as to which of the specific symptoms they experience so, a little later in this chapter, I list a variety of useful suggestions which can be included in general 'relieve anxiety scripts' as and when appropriate to the particular child. There are many scripts throughout this book that can be adapted and used as frameworks for the selected suggestions in addition to the full script that is included in this chapter. I frequently use 'Magic garden' and 'Magic bus', for younger children, and 'Thought-stopping' and 'Diminish the power of the unwanted thought' for older ones. Keep in mind that any of the scripts in Chapter 7 on anxiety would be very suitable.

In cases when there has been a precipitating traumatic incident, such as a major disaster, kidnap or burglary (and in some cases the separation anxiety may be one of a number of symptoms of Post-Traumatic Stress Disorder), it is essential at some point to address that originating experience, perhaps making use of a rewind technique or other intervention described in Chapter 7. Specific fears need to be sensitively addressed, and *credible* reassurance that is appropriate to the child's individual situation should be offered.

In many cases, however, children who develop separation anxiety will not have had any specific horrific experience and yet they seem to be unable to tolerate anything less than 100% assurance of general safety for themselves and their family. Since the truth is that none of us can be totally safe all of the time, our task, in effect, is to get them to accept that what people do (mostly unconsciously) is assess risk and then live with some degree of it. For instance, it is possible, though unlikely, that a lorry could come down my quiet cul-de-sac and run me over. However, because the chances are pretty slim that it will happen, I decide not to think about it and walk down the road with a general feeling of equanimity. Communicating this kind of idea using examples and vocabulary that are relevant to the age group – and employing a bit of humour – is actually more useful and more truthful than offering blanket reassurances of safety at all times. Sometimes, particularly when dealing with young children, merely making frequent use of the word 'safe' in your phraseology, (as in 'it's safe to sit here and relax now', and, 'we can safely say',) will be enough to bypass conscious resistance to partings from caregivers and encourage greater feelings of safety in everyday situations. (See the suggestions later in this chapter.)

Children may have ongoing problems that make it perfectly understandable for them to experience feelings of insecurity, for example, when parents divorce, when they are targets of aggression or bullying, or there has been a death or illness in the family. This type of background is not uncommon in cases of separation anxiety so it is crucial to take a full case history from the parent before the session, in addition to eliciting information from the child directly. Taking care to ensure that the parents understand what you are aiming to do will help the parents support both the child and your therapy.

Having said all of the above, I have also frequently treated children for separation anxiety who come from families that are genuinely loving, intelligent, thoughtful, well adjusted, protective (but certainly not overprotective) and that have calm dispositions. In such cases, just treat the symptoms, stay alert and remain open: you will often find extra little pieces of the jigsaw as you go along.

I have found it is helpful to give a handout to parents with ideas that they can use as a source of support when coping with their children's fears and anxieties around being separated from home and/or the parents. Parents, understandably, are often at their wit's end when the problem has been going on for some time and they have tried one approach after another, often confusing themselves as well as their children! Parents tend to welcome such a handout as long as it is offered as a suggested guideline rather than a list of regulations.

Separation Anxiety Handout: Tips for Parents and Caregivers

- Try to keep a balance between being sensitive to your child's needs and not giving in to every demand or he or she will become still more dependent on you and gain even more (unconscious) control over you and the family's activities.

- Remember that you are a human being and, try as you might to get it right, you will sometimes get it wrong. Don't beat yourself up; you are doing the best you can in what can sometimes seem like impossible circumstances.

- When leaving your child at school, remind him or her that you will be back at a certain time and try to be there earlier than you said. Make sure you are never late! If there is any possibility that you will be late, warn your child in advance. If necessary, phone and explain why you are delayed and when you will be there.

- Ask the teacher to help by greeting your child as soon as he or she enters the class and by engaging him or her in an activity with other children immediately upon arrival.

- Make your child's life boring in its regularity so that there is no more uncertainty than there has to be. This may be a little inconvenient for you but it will undoubtedly help get your child through a difficult stage and guard against extending it. Get your child up at the same time, have the same breakfast routine, leave the house at the same time, and go to school by the same route. Don't get to school too early thus causing them to hang around and wait, all the while building up anxieties.

- Try to keep partings short and sweet. Always say goodbye. Never sneak out when your child isn't looking. You want to avoid uncertainty and make sure your child trusts you to do what you say you will do.

- Explain in some detail how you will be spending your day, whether you are at work or at home, so that your child can form a mental picture of what you will be doing at any given time. You may want to make light of any journeys however.

- Tell your child frequently that you love him or her, and don't wait to be asked.

- Say that at a certain time of day or during a certain activity you will be thinking of him or her.

Scripts and Strategies in Hypnotherapy with Children © 2009 Crown House Publishing and Lynda Hudson

- Give your child a photo of you to keep during the day when you are not there.

- Try not to let your child shrink away from activities and thus become isolated. For example, go with your child to a party and explain that you will stay for the first half hour and that he or she can stay for an additional half hour (or hour) without you. Be certain to be back at the time you said. If your child seems to be content, you may want to offer the option of either staying for the last hour of the party on his or her own or leaving with you then.

- Discuss outings beforehand. Once again, try to get the balance right – don't mention them too far in advance but don't suddenly announce activities at the last moment.

- If your child doesn't want to do something without you, experiment with offering a boring alternative in a cheerful, matter-of-fact way and then be prepared to accept whichever choice he or she makes with a good grace. For example, if your child is anxious about somebody else escorting him or her to an activity, you might say, 'Choice 1: Grandma and I can both take you to your swimming class. Grandma will stay for the whole time and I can stay for 5 minutes, and pick you up again afterwards. Then we'll go back to grandma's for tea. Choice 2: you can miss the swimming and just come with me to take your brother to Cubs/Scouts and sit and wait for him and then we will go straight home.' If your child chooses to sit with you at Cubs/Scouts, don't provide rewards at the unconscious level by giving lots of attention and cuddles. Obviously, don't punish him or her by being too distant either. Perhaps you could bring something to read or have a conversation on the phone in order to reinforce the boredom of the choice.

- If you have plans to go out in the evening, be certain that the person who is looking after your child is someone trustworthy and with whom he or she feels safe. Confirm in advance the time you are leaving and the time you will be back, and make sure you stick to this. Hard though it may be, try not to respond to emotional blackmail.

- Any time your child has responded in a positive, independent way, tell him or her you are proud and then give a little special attention.

A selection of useful suggestions

Different ages

The following is a selection of suggestions that are useful when treating symptoms of separation anxiety whether or not there is a full diagnosis of the disorder. One of the central ideas to communicate is safety, however, some children are so fearful that they would not be sufficiently receptive to this idea initially. One way to address this obstacle is to bypass the conscious mind and use the word 'safe' in phrases such as:

- It's safe to sit here and relax … and you can *feel very safe* … just listening to my voice and feeling more and more comfortable.

- And feeling safe and comfortable right now you can enjoy that feeling … feeling more and more comfortable and safe as you continue to listen and relax.

- You are safe/You can know you are safe/It's safe to say/You can notice that feeling of safety growing each day/You can safely accept/It's safe for you to know that you can experience feelings of safety throughout the day/You can feel very safe knowing that mummy loves you/You can safely assume/predict that dad will be keen to see your smile when he collects you.

It is helpful to offer reassuring reminders of routine activities that the parent will be carrying out during the day. This should be done with the parent and child together and, generally speaking, the more often the reminders are repeated, the better the situation, as uncertainty is what these children find hard to tolerate.

- You will remember just what mummy is doing while you are at school.

- She will be doing the cooking while you are sitting in the classroom making sure that you will have something delicious to eat when you get home.

- At break time you remember that she is doing the filing/writing a report/doing the housework/the cooking/having a meeting with clients/talking on the telephone.

Decide specific times, such as break time and lunchtime, for child and parent to agree to exchange mental messages saying that they love each other. This could be combined with a specific anchor, such as squeezing finger and thumb together (see Chapter 7 for a discussion of anchors).

- At 11 o'clock you will *remember to squeeze your finger and thumb together* … just as you are doing right now and … as soon as you squeeze … you will *feel these wonderful feelings of safety/love/calm/confidence* because you *remember just how much your mummy loves you.*

Find ways to keep a connection with parent or caregiver during the day.

- Can you see a picture/photo of Dad? Now hold that picture in your hands … what does he look like? Is he smiling? … Can you hear him telling you how much he loves you? … And tell him you love him too … wonderful … now draw your hands up towards your chest and *take that picture into your heart* and *keep it with you all day long* … *all day long he will be with you* because you have his words inside … and because you have his smile inside … and because you know how much he loves you … *he loves you very much indeed* … *you will feel strong and happy all day long* … *each day this strong safe feeling will grow stronger and stronger wherever you are* … *at home/at school/at your friend's house.*

- Imagine an invisible string/cord that is very, very strong and attach/fix one end to you and the other end to your mum … tie it tightly but notice how stretchy it is … it just stretches and stretches as far as you want it to … nobody can see it … except you, perhaps … but you know it is there … can you feel it? … That's right … *feel that invisible string/cord joining her to you all the time you are apart* … so you know even when you are apart *there is something very strong joining you together.*

- From time to time throughout the day, your memory will remind you of every time mummy has come back to collect you and she has been perfectly safe and you have been perfectly safe … and both of you are very safe and happy all day long … you know she will always be there for you.

- You can keep a note of all the things you will tell her about when she comes to collect you … I don't know whether you will write them down or whether you will just *remember them in your head* … but I do know it is very interesting to *talk about the things you've done* … which is a good reason to *be able to go to school/to your friend's house/to your after-school club* … so you will have lots of interesting things to talk about and really *enjoy that conversation when you meet.*

- While you are waiting for these worries to *disappear completely* … one thing you can notice is that each day it becomes a little easier to *forget about those thoughts* for longer and longer each day … and while you are waiting to *forget about them completely* … you will also find that *the thoughts become weaker and weaker* so that you can *put up with them more easily* … you see … I'm not saying that you will *forget about those old worries instantly* … only that … *as that forgetting happens more and more naturally* … *you are able to deal with any thoughts* that were to pop into your mind … *deal with them more and more easily* … *you can cope with them and you can put up with them* … because they seem so much less important … and now they are so much less important … you find it so much easier to dismiss them/tell yourself they are just not true … and think of something altogether more interesting … altogether more enjoyable.

132

General suggestions for tolerating having to wait

- You will find that from now on you are able to wait for mummy/daddy to arrive and *feel very safe … feel very relaxed … feel **they** are safe …* now you have left old worries in the past … and you are feeling more and more settled and safe inside … you are happy/content to wait and think of happy things … I wonder which is your happiest thought.

- In fact the harder you were even to try to think of negative/worrying thoughts, the more impossible you would find it … from now on every time you were to think of a negative thought, *a positive thought will pop into your inventive mind* to replace it. I wonder if you knew you were so inventive or whether you will surprise yourself about just *how many positive thoughts you will find.*

- Future pacing
  As each day passes you have been becoming more and more calm and relaxed … and you have been feeling more and more confident in yourself and the world around you … I wonder whether you have noticed that you have become more able to wait more patiently … wait more calmly than before without winding yourself up … more able just to wind yourself down whenever you needed to … or whether it is merely something that you do as a matter of course now without even thinking about it at all … without even thinking about it at all.

Separation Anxiety Script: Keep your thoughts in the right place

Age range: approximately 6–12 years

With adapted vocabulary, this script would be suitable for a child of any age. If the problem is severe, you might limit your aims to one or two situations initially (for example, going to school), and only add in other activities once some progress has been made.

> You know you told me that there are some things in your life that you are very, very sure of … You told me that you are very sure you know your name … your name is (Child's Name) and you really don't have to think about that at all, do you, when I ask you your name … you are just very, very certain that your name is (Child's Name) … just as in the same way you are very, very sure you know how old you are … you are (Child's age) … exactly … so I want you to think about that for a moment and notice whereabouts inside you it is that you are so sure … you are so certain … is it in your head? … Is it in your tummy? … Is it in your chest? … Mmm interesting … now, is that a warm feeling? … Light or heavy? … Moving or still? … What colour is it? … What shape is it? … ☜ **You can have the child answer out loud or just allow him or her to experience it internally.** ☞ Great … so this is the place where you keep everything that

you are very sure about … that you are very certain of … things that you know are very true … brilliant.

Now I know that you have been keeping some of your thoughts in the right place … like your name and how old you are … but I just want you to check that you are keeping all your other thoughts in the right place too … because sometimes we get into a bit of a muddle about things and start getting worried about things just because we aren't keeping our thoughts in the right place … let's check now … let's check the thought 'I love mummy' … is that in the nice warm, round place in the middle of your tummy? … ☺ **If the child hasn't told you details about the place, just ask, 'Is that in that nice sure place inside you where your name is?'** ☺ Now let's check the thought 'mummy loves me' … great … these are all in the right place … now check this one out 'mummy is fine and safe and is coming back to collect me after school' … is that in the right place and if it's not … and I think perhaps it wasn't … just *move it in there right now … make it lovely and comfy* in that nice ☺ **Elaborate on the details if you know them.** ☺ (warm, round, pink, still) place in the middle of your tummy … and nod your head when you've done it … mmm … that's better, isn't it? … Good … now you can *feel much more certain all the time* that mummy will be safely back to collect you at the end of the school day … now let's put some others in there so that it makes a real difference to how *you can be so certain/sure that you feel safe* … and mummy feels safe … and that you can be absolutely fine the whole time you are at school/at swimming classes/at your friend's house.

☺ **Get the child to move other important thoughts that have particular relevance to the child into the 'certain place' inside. Useful thoughts would be: 'I'm okay and mum's okay/I can go to school and I will be okay all the time I'm there/I can go to sleep in my bed and be absolutely certain/sure that mummy and daddy are just downstairs/I can feel strong when I say goodbye because I'm really sure mummy is coming back/I can stay in the living room/den and feel absolutely fine even when mum is in the kitchen because I know she won't leave the house without me.'**

Having moved the thoughts into the safe, certain sure place you can begin to run through guided visualisations of the desired behaviour bringing in as many senses as possible. ☺

Fantastic … keeping all of these thoughts in that certain sure place inside … I want you to know that these safe feelings will grow stronger and stronger each day … you will grow more and more certain each day that it's safe for you to forget about those old worries and just enjoy being you … so why not have a look in your mind's eye/on your mental television screen/on your internal computer screen/into your future at how things are now with *you so strong and so certain that everything will be okay* … can you see yourself (Child's Name) saying goodbye to mum at the school gates/classroom door and running off with your friend/talking to your teacher? … Look at your face (Child's Name)! … You look really happy, don't you? … You've got a big smile on your face …

you have just checked all your thoughts are in the right/certain sure place to keep yourself feeling happy and safe all day long ... all those good thoughts and feelings are *lovely and comfy* in that nice (warm, round, pink, still) place in the middle of your tummy ... and because you *feel so strong and calm*, *you are really happy to play with your friends at break/playtime* ... look, you're joining in with all the games ... and listen to your own voice ... can you hear yourself sounding so happy and relaxed and laughing with your friends?

☺ **Review the schedule for the school day, paying particular attention to the times that are unstructured, such as breaks and lunchtime.** ☺

And before you know it, it's the end of the school day and almost time to meet mummy again ... the day has gone so much more quickly than before ... there are so many interesting/happy things you want to tell her and I'm just wondering what will be the first thing mummy notices that is a bit different about you when she catches sight of you ... I wonder if it's the happy smile on your face (Child's Name) ... or whether it's your happy voice ... or whether somehow she can tell that you have a warm, strong, safe happy feeling all over your tummy ... all the way through.

Well, you've done something amazing here today and I think you can *feel very pleased with yourself and very proud of yourself* as you *begin now* to feel your fingers wanting to wriggle about and your toes wanting to wriggle too and your arms wanting to have a really good stretch as you open your eyes and come right back here and now to the room with me ... well done.

Chapter Nine

Obsessive Thoughts and Compulsive Actions

Definition

Obsessive-compulsive disorder (OCD) is an anxiety disorder in which the sufferer experiences unwanted intrusive thoughts that run through the mind repeatedly and/or the person feels compelled to perform actions or rituals that have no reasonable basis. Often, both obsessions and compulsions are present but sometimes the problem is centred on one or the other. I am less concerned here with exact definitions of the disorder as described in Diagnostic and Statistical Manual of Mental Disorders IV (DSM-IV); rather, I want to discuss some of the types of thoughts and actions that children present with inside the hypnotherapy consulting room. This chapter aims to offer some practical ways to help children who have distressing symptoms even though they may not have a full OCD diagnosis. For an OCD diagnosis the behaviour should take up more than an hour a day or be significantly disturbing to normal daily life. Adult sufferers from OCD will recognise that their behaviour is unreasonable but this is not necessarily the case with children.

No specific genes for OCD have yet been identified but it seems that genetics probably do play some part in the onset of the disorder since it tends to run in families, in a general rather than specific way; in other words, an obsessive disposition rather than an identical obsession can be passed from parents to children. Of course, it is also true that such obsessive behaviour may be observed and learned from the parent rather than inherited genetically. We await more research, but it seems likely that the answer lies in both spheres and that both genes and learning play a part. Another line of research holds that there may be a link with reduced levels of serotonin since there is some evidence that medication that increases serotonin levels alleviates the condition to some degree. However, many do not respond to this therapy. Strep throat also may play a role in sudden onset OCD in children, suggesting that there may be a link with autoimmune problems, in which case, it has been suggested that early treatment with antibiotics may be helpful.

Obsessive compulsive thoughts and behaviours are also frequent aspects of other disorders, notably Tourette Syndrome, tic disorders, Trichotillomania, Autistic Spectrum Disorder, Body Dysmorphic Disorder and eating disorders.

There is also something known as Obsessive Compulsive Personality Disorder (OCPD), which, strangely enough, does not mean that the person has OCD as such. Instead, it points to a collection of personality traits that translate into the person tending to be rigid and inflexible, and a perfectionist in his or her thinking, as well as preoccupied with rules and lists.

Frequent Obsessive Thoughts, Urges, Images, Fears and Anxieties

- Fear that they or significant others may be harmed by normal substances (e.g., shampoo or cleaning products) around the home.

- Fear of contamination by dirt, germs or infection.

- An obsessive need for order and neatness in order to prevent something terrible from occurring.

- Obsessing on blasphemous or obscene thoughts, words or images that distress them.

- Fear that they will do something to harm others, often particularly people they love.

- A constant need to be reassured that they are safe, that they or others won't be ill/won't die or that a disaster will not occur/ has not occurred.

- Obsessive counting or preoccupation with lucky or unlucky numbers, dates or shapes.

- Preoccupation with urination and excreta.

Compulsive Actions

Compulsive actions refer to those a sufferer feels compelled to perform, usually repeatedly. Often these actions have to be carried out in very precise sequences and an exact number of times or within a certain timeframe or in a particular manner and, if interrupted, need to be restarted from the beginning. There is an underlying, sometimes overwhelming, anxiety that is only relieved by performing the action or ritual. Sometimes this anxiety is general and sometimes it is related to a specific fear, for example, a fear that a loved person might die if the action is not performed.

Frequent Compulsions and Rituals

- Excessive washing, checking or sorting things.

- Obsessive repetitive touching/tapping of objects.

- Actions associated with avoiding 'dangerous' or 'contaminating' substances (often just ordinary, harmless household substances) or compensating for having unwittingly come into contact with them.

- Excessive checking that the house and car doors are locked, and drawer and cupboard handles are straight.

- Putting on clothes in a certain order.

- Obsessive repetition of words or phrases.

- Having feet pointing in a certain direction, or possessions lined up in a specific order with nobody allowed to touch them.

- Obsessive perfectionism that leads to repeated attempts to perfect homework or not even to attempt it at all for fear of failure to achieve perfection.

The above examples may consist of single actions, a series of repeated actions or even very complicated time-consuming rituals, which frequently cause problems within the wider family. Just getting a child who has washing and checking rituals to school remotely on time can cause daily frustration and disruption to the parents and siblings as well as causing high levels of anxiety and distress in the child.

Suitable Aims for Hypnotherapy Treatment

It is always better to be cautious when discussing treatment of obsessions and compulsions with parents; management rather than complete relief of symptoms should be the focus of discussion. Clearly, you would have to monitor children for many years to be completely sure that symptoms do not recur in later life nevertheless I have treated children who, on follow up, seem to have been symptom-free for a very long time. I have found it more effective to treat OCD problems before the obsessions have taken a very strong hold, therefore, I believe it is better to treat children when young rather than assume they will 'just grow out of it', as parents are sometimes assured by others.

The Use of Direct and Indirect Suggestion

I have found that very often children will respond well to quite simple scripts that contain a mixture of direct and indirect suggestion based on changing the negative emotion attached to the thought. I will always include pseudo orientation in time (known as 'future pacing' in NLP terms), coupled with embedded commands of the child behaving naturally and normally in everyday situations where they were previously plagued by unwanted thoughts or compulsions. I always use this kind of approach with some ego strengthening as a first treatment session unless there is a compelling reason to do something different. An example of this type of script can be found in the script 'Future time capsule', and it can be readily adapted to suit almost any kind of obsessive thought or compulsion that a child might present with.

Take Away the Power of the Thought

Another useful approach suitable for a first session, or any subsequent session, is an intervention designed to take away the power of the thought (Erickson (1998) calls this 'depotentiating the thought') through various types of visual or auditory mental exercises/NLP activities, which can be carried out quite casually and conversationally while you are taking a case history. Later they can be repeated within the body of a script such as 'Diminish the power of the unwanted thought' in a slightly more formal trance state.

Method

Elicit the unwanted thought and as much information about it as possible in child-friendly language appropriate to the age. Does it come in the form of words, pictures, feelings or some combination? Is it linked with particular situations, people, actions, moods, etc.? If it is accompanied by a feeling, where is it? (Sometimes, asking the question 'how do you know when you're upset … do you know in your tummy or do you know in your head or do you know somewhere else?' will give you the answer you are looking for.)

Verbal Thought

If the thought comes in words, get the child to hear it and experiment with hearing the words in different ways, for example, ask him or her to make it louder or quieter, shouted or whispered, in a friendly way or a cross way; ask if it is sung or spoken, in a child's voice or a grown-up voice? You are only limited in your questions by your ability to think up more! After each one, get the child to hear it in his or her head and experiment to see which way sounds worse and which way sounds better. You can intersperse the conversation with remarks such as, 'Hey, I bet that sounds pretty easy to ignore now'. Keep a note of the ways the voice has the least compelling effect and make use of it with suggested changes later on in the trance state. Always include a cartoon voice, which will make it sound sillier; you are aiming to take away the power of the thought so the sillier you can get it to sound the better. Maybe the child can sing the thought to him or herself to a favourite tune. Remember that all of these things can be done internally but some children will enjoy doing them out loud, particularly if it involves shouting! You could even ask the child to shout something back at the thought such as, 'Go away you stupid thought!' Go with the child's own suggestion and be quite prepared to go with a rude one if it's offered because, if you can get the child to regard the thought as funny, you will further reduce its power. Essentially, you are giving people control over something that previously had control over them. You can have the child reach out and turn down the volume of a thought or even turn it off and get him or her to practise doing this each time the thought pops up. Use the child's own ideas as they will be more inventive, meaningful and appropriate than yours.

Visual Images

Where the thought comes as an unwanted visual image, such as imagining having a serious illness or visualising the possible disastrous consequence of failing to turn off a light switch or straighten a door handle, you can get the child to play with the images. This is useful because you are encouraging these children to face the image and stand their ground rather than believing that it is so awful or frightening that it is overwhelming and must be obeyed at all costs. By including the idea of 'let's play a game with this picture' you are also covertly illustrating how they can take control of the image rather than be at its mercy.

Just as with the verbal thoughts discussed above, it is important to establish which aspects of the picture (submodalities, in NLP terms) make it more or less frightening or compelling by experimenting with seeing it in different ways. So, ask the child to get the picture in his or her mind and then ask questions about it. Is it black and white or in colour? Is it big or small? Is it far away or right in front of your face? After each answer, have the child change it and notice if it makes it better or worse. You may end up with an image that has far less impact when the child has put it on the wall, right over there, made it smaller, coloured it yellow, turned it upside down and put it into cartoon images. You have encouraged this child to turn it into a game, which can also be played at home whenever such pictures come up. This approach allows the child to take the image or idea more light-heartedly and to establish a degree of control over it at the same time. With the use of some skilful language, you can implant the suggestion that the thought will be less likely to come or that it might not even come at all. Consider the difference between, 'You can play this game with the pictures in your mind *whenever* they come into your head' and 'You can play this game with any picture *that dares even to try* to come into your mind'.

By carrying out these types of activity conversationally, you manage to gain the appropriate information to use later (after all, there is absolutely no point in your suggesting that the child sees the picture in black and white if it makes no difference to them or even makes it worse). Further, the child may succeed in altering the power of the thought right then and there in the 5 or 10 minutes it takes and anything you do later will be purely reinforcement.

Obsessive Thoughts Script: Diminish the power of the unwanted thought

Age range: approximately 8/9 years upward

And isn't it good to know now … that if ever an unwanted thought were to try to slip into your mind … you have learned a very clever/cunning way to trick it/beat it/outsmart it so it has completely lost its power now … because you are in charge/in control of your thoughts now … so I want you to know that at any time … at any place … ☺ **You can mention any specific times, places or situations in which these thoughts typically occur.** ☺ you are able to change the thought so that it really has no power over you at all … brilliant … you can do it right now … imagine some thought that you would like to change … nod your head when you've got it … and hear it in an ordinary way and then … reach out for that remote control and change the voice … that's it … (just as we did before) put it into a tiny, mousy, squeaky voice/a 'loser' cartoon character and *notice how it sounds so silly/ridiculous now* … it's the kind of voice that *you really can't take seriously* … it actually can make *you want to laugh* when you really realise now just how very stupid it was … and as *you really can't take it seriously any more* … why don't you adjust the volume

143

control and turn the sound down so it gets quieter and quieter ... that's it ... quieter and quieter so you can hardly hear it ... *you're hardly aware of it at all* ... you're hardly aware of that thought at all ... and it is so good to know that you always have your mental remote control with you so you can *make whatever changes you want to make* at any time ... at any place ... whether you're with other people or on your own ... you will always remember that you have your remote control so you are in complete control ... amazing ... well done ... you are so good at this.

And now you've got the hang of changing that silly/pathetic old voice ... you will find it totally easy to change the picture in your mind too ... let's do one now ... get up a picture of some old thought that used to worry you ... ☟ **You can mention any scenario the child told you about before.** ☟ that's it ... nod your head when you've got it ... well done ... now (just as we did before) ... first of all put it right over there ... about as far away as the wall ... and as you do ... notice how much easier it is to *stay calm* when you look at it ... and now begin to change the colours in the picture to the calmest ones you can imagine right now ... and you can imagine so well ... that's it ... now ... feeling very calm and very relaxed ... as you look at that picture ... notice how the colours are fading right away ... let them fade away completely so that the whole picture becomes transparent ... you can see right through it ... amazing ... and now notice how soon a different picture comes through of you looking so happy, looking so relaxed and so positive ... and you are just ignoring that old thought and getting on with what you prefer to do ... look at that confident look on your face as you know so well deep down that it's fine for you to *forget about that old thing* more and more every day ... in fact as each day goes by you will *find it harder and harder* to remember that old thing ... actually the harder you were to try to remember it, the more you would forget it ... you will either forget to remember it or remember to forget it ... and wonder whether that forgetting is the same as not remembering ... or will you just prefer to *forget about the whole thing* because you have just left it in the past where it belongs ... just like you left other things in the past ... like when you were a toddler and learning to walk and used to fall over and pick yourself up ... I don't suppose you ever think of that at all ... you just left it all in the past with the other things you've forgotten about ... so in a few moments time I'm going to ask you to come zooming back in your mind to the room here with me ... remembering that you feel positive and confident and strong ... and at the count of 8 you will open your eyes (if they have been shut) and at the count of 10 you will be feeling full of energy ... maybe wanting to wriggle about and have a stretch ... ready to go home and enjoy the rest of your day.

Obsessive Thoughts Script: Future time capsule

Age range: approximately 8–12 years

This script uses direct suggestions and a guided visualisation, including embedded commands, of a future time when all problems have been resolved.

And (Child's Name) as you are feeling so comfy and relaxed right now … I want you to know that as each day goes by you will become more and more relaxed in your mind … and you will *feel so relaxed* that if any unwanted thought were to even try to pop into your mind … it wouldn't bother you at all … it would *have no importance to you at all* in fact … the harder you were to even try to get worried in that same old way … *the more impossible it would be for you to be bothered at all* … in fact you *hardly notice those old thoughts at all* … you *become so relaxed* … and *become so confident* … you can just shrug your shoulders and find … as the days and the weeks go speeding by now … *those old thoughts just seem to drop away into the past* where they belong … less and less important … until *now they have no importance at all*.

And right now it's time to go on a journey into your imagination … I'd like you to climb into that time capsule over there and zoom into the future where *that old problem has been completely solved* … go far enough so there isn't the slightest bit of it left … and nod your head when you're there … and just look out of your capsule window and take a look at (Child's Name) without a care in the world.

That's it … well done … now just enjoy being here with (Child's Name) where everything is sorted out … right now … here and now … now and then … sooner and later … *you are confident and relaxed and in charge of your thoughts* … now you *only think about things that you like to think about* … your mind thinks positive thoughts … you *choose to think comfortable thoughts* and you are very comfortable with those thoughts … *you are in complete control of your thoughts now.*

☞ **At this point, talk the child through some scenarios in which he or she used to be particularly bothered by unwelcome thoughts but is now calm and unworried and thinking positively instead. The following is an example of a child who was obsessed by fear of contamination when anybody used cleaning materials and when he was asked to use bath or shower products. You will notice that the child is being asked to hop in and out of the picture; this is to give more repetitions of the positive experience and also to change the dynamics of the response. For some people, the experience of looking at themselves as though in a movie is powerful, whereas others respond more strongly to feeling themselves to be in the experience now.** ☞

Look at you … you are amazingly cool … there you are in the kitchen … just sitting at the kitchen table and your mum is cleaning up the sink … she's done the washing up … and look she's wiping the table and you aren't taking any notice of her at all …

(By the way, maybe next time you can offer to help her!) … You are getting on with your homework … *happy* that the table is *clean* and you can *safely* keep your books *nice and clean and tidy* … your mind is clear … *you are thinking clearly and calmly* and *you look so confident* … look at you … what lets you *know that you are so confident now?* Is it the laid-back look on your face? … Is it that *your whole body is sooo relaxed and calm?* Great, you are doing this so well … hop out of your time capsule now and actually be there and feel those confident calm relaxed feelings … notice where they are in your body … in your head … as you are there totally in control of your thoughts while all that cleaning is going on … well done … fantastic.

So hop back into your capsule and take another look at the situation in the bathroom … is that you taking a shower … choosing which shower gel to use? … washing your hair without a care in the world … fantastic … *everything is so much easier now* … and I wonder how you knew that the best thing for you was to sing to yourself in the shower to increase your feelings of confidence and control … did it just come to you all in a flash? … Or did the idea creep up on you a little bit at a time? … Whichever way it was … congratulations for finding the best way for you to *really enjoy using the bathroom now.*

So once again jump out of your time capsule for a moment or two … and just be there now … feel the warm water on your skin … … *feel how good it is … feel how confident and relaxed you are* … and *it's safe* to feel that relaxed, calm feeling as you smooth on the shower gel … it's so soothing on your skin, is it not? … Soft and soothing and *safe to use* … and this can *feel so good* … let's do it again … doing it in half the time this time … as though you are in a fast forward movie … that's it … now do it one more time … wonderful … and enjoying just a few moments more here … before I ask you to jump back into the time capsule only as quickly as you can store all those safe bathroom feelings inside you … and zoom back to the present moment with all those wonderful, calm, confident feelings safely stored inside you … so you can feel those wonderful safe and calm, clean feelings all the way through.

So, zooming back … all the way back … feeling a whoosh of energy coming back into your body so that your fingers and your toes feel they want to wriggle about … your arms want to have a really good stretch and your eyes are open wide and you feel amazingly good … amazingly calm … amazingly in control.

Obsessive Thoughts Script: Thought-stopping on your computer mind

Age range: approximately 12 years upward (if they are keen computer users, you can adapt the language accordingly and use it with younger children too)

The script uses some ideas from cognitive therapy, e.g., thought-stopping and replacing negative thoughts with positive ones and is based on the same concept and format of the script 'STOP messages on your computer mind' in Chapter 3.

A useful way to think about our brains is that they are rather like computers only far more impressive … so I want you to imagine right now that *you can* … go into your mind computer and click on the *Stop Unwanted Thoughts* program … can you see the window come up? … That's right … now (Child's Name) just have a look and see if it is running properly … sometimes what happens is that there are little errors in the program that stop it from working properly … for example, some people find that the program has been allowing false thoughts to come in.

You told me that you had sometimes been getting thoughts in your head that stopped you from doing things/caused you to keep touching certain objects over and over, didn't you? … Now I want you to *understand fully that … that thought is completely untrue* … and *doesn't belong in that program at all* … so I want you to click on the delete button and *clear that thought immediately* … good, excellent … wasn't that satisfying! … The next thing to do is to set a reminder message so that … if ever that false thought were to come into your head again … a big stop sign will come up in your mind … it's a big red sign with STOP written on it … can you see it? Make it bright, bright red … make it very big indeed … and listen, it has a very loud voice like this … STOP! THIS IS AN ERROR MESSAGE FROM YOUR STOP UNWANTED THOUGHTS PROGRAM … FALSE THOUGHT HAS SLIPPED THROUGH … DELETE PLEASE …DELETE PLEASE … and then you hit the delete key … and because *you (Child's Name) are definitely clever/intelligent/bright enough* to know the difference between a false thought and a true thought … (you are *more* than clever enough) … you can type in a true thought in place of that old false one … *for example … it's perfectly safe to touch the waste bin/walk near the rubbish bin … so just do that now and nod your head when you've done it.* ☺ **Include any suggestions that are appropriate for the child in question.** ☺ Keep typing … it doesn't affect me at all … it can't possibly harm me … it was just a false thought/computer virus in the *Stop Unwanted Thoughts* program. ☺ **Don't use the word virus if they have obsessive thoughts about illness!** ☺ Now practise saying this: 'It was just a false thought. It's perfectly safe *to touch the waste bin/walk near the rubbish bin/to only wash your hands once/turn the switch off without checking it/say that name'* to yourself in your strongest, most confident voice … that's right … now do it again but do it louder this time … brilliant … hear how good that sounds … get a feel of that confidence … isn't it great? … And each time you *change the thought* you will *become calmer, more confident and more in control each day.*

Now before you finish, go and have a look for any other possible false thoughts … or any other silly errors that may be stopping the program from running properly. ☺ **Here you can refer to anything that the child may have told you about in the pre-trance discussion.** ☺

Delete everything that is not useful or is harmful to you and type in something that will make your program work better, for example … *I am a positive person, I am calm and I am confident* … *I know the difference between true and false* … add any positive message that's right for you and now save that information and close the program … nod your head when you've done it.

☺ **Pause long enough for the child to do this. Watch his or her fingers – you can often see movements as the positive messages are typed.** ☺

Excellent … now your brain can run your *Stop Unwanted Thoughts* program properly and each day as you *practise doing everything calmly and confidently* … *you increase your confidence daily.* ☺ **Have the child visualise being in everyday situations with the unwanted thought program error-free so that he or she is deleting any false thoughts that come in and replacing them with true ones.** ☺

Great, so now that the program is running really well, I'd like you to click on to the screen where your program is funtioning perfectly … look at you … you are looking so calm and confident … as you get on with the everyday things in your life in such a positive way … look at you … you've just finished an apple and you're walking over to the bin … hey … see how you're throwing the core in the bin and you feel perfectly fine … and *you know it's safe* for you to *feel fine now as you walk right up to the bin* and you throw all the unwanted stuff in the bin … by the way, you can throw thoughts in there too if you like … don't *you look calm and in control*?

And listen … is that your mum asking you to bring the bin downstairs so she can empty it? … and as soon as a negative voice starts in your head … the moment it begins … listen … there's a message coming in loud and clear … STOP! THIS IS AN ERROR MESSAGE FROM YOUR 'STOP UNWANTED THOUGHTS' PROGRAM … FALSE THOUGHT HAS SLIPPED THROUGH … DELETE PLEASE …DELETE PLEASE … And then you hit the delete key in double quick time … give yourself a true thought … a useful thought … and you know you are perfectly fine … nothing bad will happen … you can do this … you are in control … you will do this … and I wonder (Child's Name) who is most surprised … is it your dad or your mum?… as they see you coming downstairs just holding that bin without a care in the world … look at their faces … how proud are they? … How proud are *you* … that you have got your thought program working so well?

Great … in a few moments time I am going to ask you to come zooming back in your mind to the room when I count from 1 to 10 … but just before I do … I'd like you to see those positive situations over in your mind another five times very, very quickly … ೨ **Describe them briefly to be sure the child is using the scenarios previously referred to.** ೨ just quickly enough to get them fixed into your mind so that no old unwanted thought can ever have that power over you again. ೨ **Pause long enough for the child to do this and then count to 10 to reorient him or her to the room.** ೨

Compulsive Actions Script: Wait before you act

Age range: approximately 10 years upward

The script uses a combination of reframing and a mild behavioural modification technique. It offers two 'future pacing' visualisation options; one with the use of a coping mechanism of waiting before performing the compulsive action and one with simply no desire to perform the action at all.

Use the 'Find the right place' induction in Chapter 2 or have them drift off to any favourite place.

I want you to know that here in this special place where you can *feel very comfortable … feel very comfortable with yourself in every way …* you can use your fantastic inner mind to do some amazing things … I don't know whether you already know or whether this will be new to you that the main job of your inner mind is to *keep you safe and to protect you …* and sometimes it dreams up unusual ways to help you *feel safe …* and at a time when you were younger when … for one reason or another you were a bit anxious or unsettled … I believe that your inner mind dreamed up a funny way to help you by doing something like … touching something for luck/double checking you've done something/making sure your hands were clean … it kind of made you feel you had some control over what was happening in your life … although of course … it was only a *feeling* of control and it wasn't really true … but still … it did help you for a bit at the time and then the whole thing got rather out of hand, didn't it … it seemed to take over … but now … you know that you not only *NEED to change things … you really WANT to change things … you really want to change this old touching (washing/pulling/checking) habit … so y*ou can talk to your special inner mind and ask it to help you … *make some wonderful changes …* now … you can ask it to help you reprogram your thinking and feeling in just the way you like … you can feel totally calm and comfortable all over … all the way through … you can talk very quietly in your head so it's only your inner mind that hears you … so just nod your head when you are ready to begin … that's right … so … first of all say thank you Inner Mind for trying to help protect me and keep me safe. ೨ **Leave enough time in the pauses for the child to repeat or rephrase your words in his or her mind. You can add encouragements as appropriate.** ೨ Good … and now explain that this old touching (washing/pulling/checking) is not helping you any more … in fact it is making you feel quite uncomfortable/bad instead ... just use your own words to explain how bad that habit is making you feel ... nod your head when you've done it ... that's it ... now explain that you would really like its help to *become more relaxed and more in control* ... ask it if it will help you here ... today ... to begin to *get back your own control* and *put an end to that old habit* ... and nod your head when it agrees ...that's great ... so now your special inner mind truly understands what a pain/what a problem/how difficult all this has been for you ... it will dream up a way for you to *feel naturally more calm and confident* on the inside so there will be absolutely no need for all that old touching (washing/pulling/checking) to feel safe ... because you *WILL* feel safe ... you *WILL know you are safe deep down inside* ... you *WILL know you are calm* ... and because you know you are calm and you know you are safe ... all those old boring *habits will begin to fade away* ... *fade away* until you are not aware of them any more ... and as they are fading ... you will find that in all those situations where once you used to feel you had to touch (wash/pull/check) several times ... you will know that you can easily wait before you do it ... You can wait 5/10/20 minutes before you touch (wash/pull/check) ... you will find that you can easily resist ... it's so much easier now ... You can *wait a little longer* and *wait a little longer still* and *wait a lot longer* ... and *know you are fine while you wait* ... and while you are waiting you may *have a very strong urge to go and have a drink of water* ... and while you drink the water you dilute all old unwanted urges ... with each sip you can feel them becoming less and less strong ... they become weaker and weaker ... and as they become weaker ... *you become stronger* ... and altogether you *feel more and more calm and relaxed* ... and as you feel more and more relaxed ... your confidence is increasing ... so I am not sure just how amazingly quickly you find that you can *cut down that old habit by a quarter* and then by a half ... or will you *cut down by a half straightaway*? ... and of course ... you will find that the urge becomes weaker and weaker ... and then the urge comes less and less often ... or does that happen at just the same time? ... At just the same time as you *become generally more confident in yourself* and *happier in your everyday life* ... at home, at school wherever you are.

☾ At this point, if the habit has been very strong or seems to be a bit resistant, you may want to include some future pacing of the coping mechanism; a guided visualisation of the child waiting 5 minutes and then 10 minutes and then 15 minutes, etc., before performing the action or going for a glass of water and becoming gradually more in control every day. But if the habit is already reasonably weak, you may prefer to move straight on to Option 2, the successful visualisation of there being no trace of the habit at all. ☾

Future pacing: Option 1

Now ... there are different ways that this might happen and I am not quite sure whether that fading will happen little by little by a lot ... or whether it *will happen immediately all at once* ... let's zoom forward in time to see it happen little by little by a lot ... can you notice in your mind's eye that you are there by

the front door ... you've just come in ... there is ... at first ... a tiny little bit of that old urge left but you are so much stronger than before ... you know you can resist that old urge ... listen to yourself telling yourself that you can wait ... there's really no need to touch it for the moment ... you are fine ... look how calm and relaxed you are ... but you decide to go and get that glass of water and let that little bit of feeling get less and less ... get weaker and weaker as the feeling dilutes ... that old feeling gets weaker and weaker ... and as you finish the water look how you are feeling strong enough to go straight upstairs to your bedroom/into the living room/to use your computer/get started on your work/read a book ... well done ... absolutely great ... you are doing so well ... you are amazing ... are you amazing yourself just how brilliantly you are doing?
 ꙮ **Include some more typical scenarios that you have already discussed showing how the urge gets weaker and weaker.** ꙮ

Future pacing: Option 2

Now zoom forward in time right into the way *it might happen all in one go* ... all at once ... *all* of those old urges have faded away ... just disappeared ... not part of your life any more ... *you have absolutely no wish to touch in that same old way* ... you have absolutely no desire to do it ... *no urge to do that old thing any more* ... so just look at you superstar ... there you are ... you've just come in though the front door ... you keep going straight on to the kitchen/bedroom/dining room ... you look so comfortable and at ease ... your mind is on your football match/new game/computer/TV programme/other favourite activity ... you are calm, relaxed and in control ... look at your face ... so happy and smiley ... feel how at ease your body is ... hear the way you're chatting in such a relaxed way to your mum ... and look at her face and notice how proud she is of you ... really great ... you really are a superstar.

Trichotillomania in Children

Trichotillomania belongs to a group of disorders called Body Focused Repetitive Behaviours (BFRBs). Others include skin picking, nail biting, mouth chewing, nose scratching or picking, and foot tapping.

Trichotillomania is sometimes called Trich or TTM.

Symptoms include pulling/picking/rubbing or fiddling with hair usually from the scalp, eyelashes or eyebrows but it can be from any area of the body.

There is a strong build-up of tension or anxiety prior to picking or pulling that seems only to be relieved by plucking the hair out. The tension may be experienced as emotional anxiety or as a physical sensation such as an itch, or both at the same time.

Once pulled out, the hair may be further examined, played with or quite often chewed or eaten. Long-term eating of hair (Trichophagia) can cause hairballs (Trichobezoars) in the stomach or small intestines, which, in extreme cases, may need to be surgically removed.

This relief and pleasurable or comforting sensation is usually only temporary and is followed by more tension and guilty feelings for having given in to the urge. It is nearly always accompanied by embarrassment, shame or feelings of isolation with a strong need to hide both the habit and the effects from others.

The action may be carried out consciously or unconsciously, or often both on different occasions.

When done consciously there may be an urge to find just the right type of hair to pull; it may be longer, thicker, more prominent or in a particular area for example.

The behaviour is often performed in private and is frequently denied.

Onset commonly occurs around 10 years of age or in the early teens, but it can also be seen in younger children.

In babies, playing and twisting the hair is usually comfort behaviour.

In toddlers, it is normally just a continuation of a comfort habit.

From about 3 years of age it could also be one among a range of tantrum behaviours. Subsequently, if the child notices the parent reacting to the hair pulling, it may become an attention-seeking device.

From about 5 years old, TTM may still be the continuation of a straightforward habit or angry/tantrum behaviour. It may also be a symptom of stress or emotional upset, particularly if it has a sudden onset. You should check for stressors in the home or school environment. The pulling can be a way of expressing unhappy or angry feelings that the child finds hard to articulate.

Trichotillomania is seen in response to stressful or upsetting situations, but it also can be a response to tiredness and boredom. It can be a way for children to distract themselves from distressing events or thoughts.

Children who have TTM may also display other obsessive-compulsive behaviours.

It is more frequently found in girls (and women) than in boys (and men). Reports of the incidence of TTM vary considerably and this may be in part due to the fact that the behaviour is so frequently denied that it is difficult to collect reliable data. Reports of between 2% and 10% of the population have been quoted.

In young children, it may be thought of more as a short-term habit disorder; however, because TTM in older children and adults can last for weeks, years or decades, it is prudent to treat it early.

Antidepressant medications (selective serotonin reuptake inhibitors [SSRIs]) are sometimes used to reduce the impulse to pull but generally they are not recommended for use with children.

Appropriate Treatment Aims for Hypnotherapy

- Relaxation and reduction of anxiety.
- Coping strategies for stress and negative emotions.
- Coping strategies for resisting temptation to carry out the activity.
- Distraction from the activity.
- Elimination or reduction of the habit.
- Coping strategies for dealing with the consequences, such as embarrassment or guilt.
- Confidence and self-esteem building.

All the scripts given earlier in this chapter would be suitable for use with Trichotillomania. The hand levitation script that follows is particularly useful to include at some point in the treatment, perhaps in the second session. The first benefit is that it is such a powerful convincer and the second is that it makes use of the already-established action of the hand rising towards the head. I would probably not use it in a first treatment session simply because I normally point out at the initial session or to parents before treatment even commences that clinical hypnosis is nothing like stage hypnosis, and I am aware that this technique might be interpreted as being somewhat 'stagy'. It does work wonderfully well, however, and particularly so with teenagers.

Trichotillomania hand levitation script

Age range: approximately 10 years upward

(The child needs to be mature enough to distinguish between deliberate conscious and unconscious lifting of the hand.)

The script uses a combination of dissociation and reframing indirect and direct suggestion.

> I'd like you to place your hands very, very lightly on your legs, just like this … that's right … so lightly that your fingertips are only just touching your legs ℘ **Demonstrate on your own lap rather than touch the child.** ℘ and as you *fix your eyes on the hand* that used to pull at your hair … let yourself notice … *really notice I mean* … how the hand gets rather fuzzy and blurred as you keep looking … that's it … and as you *look really hard* … are you noticing I wonder that you *begin to feel that fuzzy and blurred feeling in your fingers* too? … A fuzzy feeling that feels light … so light that the fingers begin to feel light as a feather … so light … as if they can float … *they can float* … and maybe it's just one finger … or two or three … that start to float up all on their own … lifting up off your lap … some children/people tell me they even imagine that *balloons are pulling the hand up higher and higher* … they even *see the balloons pulling the hand higher and higher.* ℘ **Remember that there are many children who have a strong dislike or fear of balloons so leave out this imagery if it is not appropriate.** ℘ And that lovely light feeling floats back into your wrist … yes … and all the way back into your arm … keep looking as that hand floats higher and higher as if it were going towards your head … but look now as it is stopping … stopping … stopped completely and ℘ **If you feel the child would be comfortable, proceed to eye closure, but if not, just leave him or her with eyes open.** ℘ if you *close your eyes now* you can still see that hand there in front of your eyes and I would like you know that you can … *have a conversation in your head* with that special part of you that *is truly in control of your hand now* … ask it to *stay in control/in charge of your hand* even when you might have forgotten to *stay in control/in charge* … ask it to *keep so much in control* that it never lets it go to your hair/eyebrows/eyelashes to pull them

ever again … brilliant … that's right … explain that you really want to leave your hair alone now so that it grows back strong and thick just like *you want it to grow back* … good … that's it … now nod your head when you've done it … wonderful … and I want you to notice that when you *begin to feel that hand getting heavy again … you will know that special part of you has given you your answer … you will know deep down inside … that from now on you are in perfect control of your hands and fingers …* and as *your hand is getting so heavy* that it is just sinking down on to your lap … you will *feel a wonderful sense of calm and relaxation …* you might even begin to *feel a little bit sleepy as your hand touches your lap …* and notice how your whole body feels comfortable, calm and relaxed … and as you *enjoy that lovely calm and relaxed feeling …* can you *notice that great, confident feeling you get in your mind*? … A wonderful confident feeling that lets you *know that you are in control of that old habit now …* and *this confident control will grow stronger and stronger every day* … you will find that you *feel so good in yourself … so calm in your mind … so confident in yourself* that you can *deal with any cross/angry/annoying/irritating/frustrating/sad/unhappy/bored feeling … deal calmly and confidently with any situation that happens at school … deal calmly and confidently with any situation that happens at home* and isn't it amazing to notice that you *have absolutely no urge to pull or pick your hair/eyelashes/eyebrows at all.*

Fantastic … and just before we finish and you find that your hands and fingers and arms are absolutely and completely their normal weight … not too heavy and not too light … you get some mental pictures of you looking so pleased with yourself that you *have* managed to leave your hair alone when you are watching television … that yo*u are feeling so calm and confident now when you do your homework …* your mum is telling you *how amazing you are* that you have *cut down/cut out that old habit so well …* that you are feeling so relaxed in bed that you *drift comfortably and calmly off to sleep and your hands are absolutely nowhere near your head …* amazing … fantastic … well done.

And now it really is time to wake up feeling all the energy coming back into your body … your fingers wanting to wriggle around as I count from 1 to 10 … feeling they want to stretch … you want to stretch all over … well done … back here … and your arms, hands and fingers are feeling absolutely normal … completely their normal weight.

Chapter Ten

Sleeping Difficulties

Common Sleep Problems and Ways to Work with Them

There are many different kinds of sleep problems encountered by children. Most have accompanying or underlying anxiety, and tend to fall into the categories outlined below. As I discuss the issues, I will point to a suitable script, which will follow later in the chapter.

Worrying Thoughts and Feelings

The child has worrying thoughts and feelings that either keep him or her from falling asleep or that prevent him or her from going back to sleep upon waking in the middle of the night.

Sometimes the problem is not really a 'sleep problem'; rather it is the expression of anxieties a child may have managed to suppress during the day while involved in other activities. The quiet time in bed before sleep allows these anxieties to surface (in the same way as it does with adults). In this case, the treatment should be directed at the real source of the problem and it is useful to speak to the parent on the telephone in advance to discover more about the background. It is important to find out how long the problem has been in existence and what was happening in their lives when the sleeping difficulties first arose. If there has been 'sudden onset sleeping difficulty', it is probable that the cause will be anxiety or an emotional upset rather than a sleeping disorder in its own right. Although I like to discover as much information as I can in advance, I bear in mind that the parent's eye view may be different from that of the child so I always ask the child directly during the session about what was going on when he or she first started finding it a bit hard to get to sleep. Find out what makes it worse and what makes it better. Sometimes, especially with girls, an argument at school or being dropped by a so-called best friend may be deeply upsetting and more difficult for them to deal with than something more obvious and serious as far as the parent is concerned.

Sleep is sometimes associated with death, anaesthesia or illness by the child when these have occurred in the recent, or sometimes not so recent, past. When a grandparent, for example, has died, and the child has not been given an adequate explanation of what has happened either because the parents are trying to protect him or her from pain or because they have oversimplified what happens when someone dies, an association between sleep and death may inadvertently result. Euphemisms such as 'put to sleep' when a pet dies can cause children to fear sleep lest they might suffer the same fate! These fears need to be gently elicited so that specific, direct and indirect suggestions for reassurance and safety can be given, which usually helps enormously. If you suspect that such fears exist but remain unspoken, you can include presuppositions of safety and the certainty of waking up in the morning in your 'wake-up procedure' whatever the main thrust of the session – 'after you have slept safely all through the night ... every night ... you will wake up every morning wide awake and looking forward to the day'.

Always take care when using 'sky type' inductions because children might have associations with somebody who has died having gone to heaven in the sky. This is information that you can find out from the parent in advance.

Elicit children's bedtime thoughts

When you go to bed what are you thinking about which helps you to feel happy/safe/strong/brave/calm? (Almost certainly they will tell you they are not doing this, but this question gives you information you need and also helps to point out that changing their thinking would be a useful thing to do.)

When you go to bed what are you thinking about when you're feeling anxious/unhappy/sad? (If/when they give you this answer, they are providing information from which to choose an intervention or formulate your suggestions.)

Let's play detective: what makes it worse? What makes it better?

Move them towards a solution:

So, how would it be if you were to think about the things that help you to feel happy at bedtime and only think about the other things in the daytime when you feel stronger and can deal with them in a positive way? Would that be helpful? How about I help you to do that? Great, tell me some of the things that make you feel happy/relaxed.

A suitable script would be 'Deal with unwanted night-time thoughts', but before using it, talk about the worrying thoughts themselves and help the child to reframe them or use one of the methods in Chapter 7 on anxiety. Then use the sleeping script and reinforce the reframe within the trance state as appropriate. Incidentally, as the script includes a suggestion to write down or draw the worrying thought, you might also want to encourage children to do this in reality before they go to sleep, telling them to look at it again in the daytime when they are more able to deal with it resourcefully. This has the effect of externalising the thoughts and allowing the unconscious mind to let go of the anxiety.

Summary: Dealing with Unwanted Night-time Thoughts

- Get background information from parents beforehand about current circumstances.
- Elicit bedtime thoughts.
- Reframe where possible.
- Use suggestions for externalisation of worries.
- Use suggestions for safety where appropriate.
- Guided visualisation of child relaxed, calm and able to sleep quite happily.
- Suitable script: 'Deal with unwanted night-time thoughts'.

Sounds

The child is either kept awake or is awakened by sounds in or outside the house such as heating/water pipes/floorboards creaking/trains/traffic.

It is important to get to the root of why these sounds cause a problem since, in my experience, it is rarely simply that the sound itself disturbs. If the latter *is* the case, just give suggestions for changing the focus of attention and use the sounds for triggers of relaxation; generally though, it is more likely that children think the sounds are being made by burglars, monsters, or something frightening out of a television programme or computer game. It might be that the noises sound vaguely spooky and disturbing. It is important to describe and explain the processes behind the sounds and reframe them as normal and follow this with direct suggestions for the sounds being of no importance to them at all. Conversely and paradoxically you can give suggestions for using the sounds as triggers to turn over and sleep more deeply. Include a guided visualisation of the child sleeping through sounds and if he or she should be roused, saying, 'Oh, it's only the pipes; that's fine. I can go back to sleep' or 'It's just the stairs having a conversation'.

Generally it is good to make suggestions for safety, calm and relaxation, but you always have to use your judgment. Blanket suggestions for safety could be inappropriate depending on the domestic situation or when there has, in fact, been a burglary. In these instances, you need to confer with the parents first regarding what has been done to make the environment safer.

Summary: Dealing with Night Sounds

- Elicit fears.
- Explain and reframe where possible.
- Use suggestions for selective attention.
- Use the sounds as triggers for relaxation, calm and sleep.
- Guided visualisation of child relaxed, calm and able to sleep amidst the sounds.
- Suitable script: 'Sounds don't bother you at all'.

The Child is Frightened of the Dark

The following may sound strange, and as if it would go without saying, but it is a good idea to talk to both parent and child and suggest that it is okay to leave the light on in the room or on the landing so that the child can feel comfortable. It is surprising how often it seems that this simple solution has been overlooked! At the very least there should be a bedside lamp and easy access to a light switch so the child can put it on whenever necessary. Again, it sounds obvious but in order to deal with the fear itself, you need to find out what the child is afraid might happen and this is not always as straightforward as it seems. Sometimes children do not want to appear 'babyish' and so are not always very forthcoming about their actual fears. Here are some suggested questions to help circumvent this issue.

> **Find Out What They Fear Can Happen in the Dark**
>
> • Show a comic strip depicting a frightened cartoon character in bed and ask, 'What do you think this character could be frightened of?'
>
> • What is the craziest thing a child could be frightened of? (Repeat this question substituting 'most unusual', 'funniest', and finishing with 'most likely'.)
>
> • Lots of people are frightened of the dark at different stages during their life; what do you think the most likely thing is at age 5/age 8/age 10, etc.? DON'T start with the child's own age group.
>
> • Suitable script: Selection of 'Suggestions for Fear of the Dark'.

If you obtain information about a specific fear, obviously you will choose a script or intervention most appropriate to the individual case. Look for ideas in Chapter 7 on anxiety.

Fear of Monsters or Other Spooky Creatures

Use cartoon imagery to befriend the monster or cut it down to size. Change the black colour to pink with yellow spots. Add wellington boots, funny hats, etc. Do all of this in an interactive, conversational way pre-trance and have the child repeat it when in a more relaxed trance state to reinforce the effect. Doing it in an interactive, conversational way first allows you to explore what works best for the particular child and also shows the child that he or she can change the internal pictures and be in control of thoughts.

So, how big is this monster? Oh, *that* big … what if you make him even bigger? Does that make him better or worse? Now let's make him smaller. Does that make him better or worse? Okay, you like him better when he's smaller. Okay, let's make him a bit smaller still then. Great! Now let's see what he looks like if you make him pink with green stripes. Is that better or worse than having him be pink with yellow spots? Oh, so you like him with green stripes! What sort of face does he have? Suppose we make him look a bit like Shrek? Do you like him better this way?

Helping children to be as inventive and involved in the process as possible will make it more likely that they can do it on their own in their bedroom. Reframe whenever you can as above – getting them to agree that the monster looks better smaller by saying something like, 'Oh, so you like him better this way'. With this type of statement, you are actually getting them to agree that they like him rather than being frightened by him. Follow with any suitable relaxing sleeping script and include reminders that they can change the pictures in their mind whenever they want to do so.

Summary: Dealing with Monsters

- Elicit fears.
- Reframe when possible.
- Use humour whenever possible.
- Use any intervention that gives the child control – changing the size, colour, proximity of the picture of a monster in his or her mind.

- Use cartoon imagery, making characters friendly and dressing them up in funny clothes, etc.

- Use guided visualisations of the child relaxed, calm and able to laugh at old thoughts.

- Suitable scripts: Choose extracts from any scripts in this chapter and also from scripts in Chapter 7 on anxiety.

Disturbing Dreams/Nightmares

Recent research on dreaming by Joe Griffin and Ivan Tyrrell (2003) proposes that a 'function of dreams is a metaphorical acting out of undischarged, emotional arousal from our unfulfilled (conscious) expectations of the previous day'. If we accept this view, it may be the case that the dream prevents the brain from being overloaded and can bring about satisfactory closure to the worries of the day and so be a positive event. However, children are more likely to be brought to see you because their sleep is disturbed by frequent, disturbing dreams or recurring nightmares so it clearly makes sense to try to uncover what has been going on recently and what their daytime thoughts might be. Ideally it is best to get the child to talk about this and reframe worries and concerns in your preceding talk, although, of course, this may be easier said than done! However, as we know with adults, merely being given the opportunity to express concerns, be listened to and be taken seriously can be enormously helpful; it is no less true with children.

When nightmares are frequent and disruptive, children may become afraid to go to sleep or may awaken distressed during the night. Obviously, this is a problem in and of itself, but it also can set up a habit of poor sleeping patterns. If it is a recurring dream, children will usually be able to describe it to you and, depending on the age, you can ask them what they make of the dream. Even if they can't put it into words or don't want to do so, you will be able to use a rewind technique without necessarily knowing the content yourself.

Rewind Technique

If there is a known causal upsetting event such as an accident, a bullying incident (also see Chapter 11), a scary television programme
or a turbulent plane journey, I often use a rewind technique on the
actual event first and then I deal with the dream sequence, particularly if it is a recurring dream. The recurring nature of the dream
suggests that the incident itself has not been adequately addressed
or processed so the fear remains unresolved. If no causal event
is discovered, you can use the rewind technique on the dream
sequence itself. See Chapter 7 on anxiety for the description of the
technique.

Explain that you are going to show the child how to remember
the event in a way that will no longer be frightening. This can be
done either in a conversational and interactive way or by taking
the child into a more relaxed trance state in which first you get him
or her to imagine drifting off to a favourite place where he or she
feels safe and resourceful. Have the child re-dream the nightmare
on an imaginary TV screen (an example of dissociation) and do the
rewind technique, including the use of bright colours and cartoon
characters if appropriate.

Change the Dream

After going through the rewind procedure, get the child to imagine
seeing the dream on a TV screen exactly as he or she would have
preferred it to happen. Maybe the child is strong and calm throughout, maybe he is twice his normal size, maybe she has a good laugh
or responds with a clever quip, or maybe he can run away instead
of being frozen to the spot, or maybe the ending is changed so that
the child emerges in control rather than as the victim of the situation. Have the child see it through and check if there are any more
positive changes that should be made. Continue making further
changes until the child is happy with the result. Include embedded
commands for calm, coping and control wherever appropriate as
you go along. Once the child is completely satisfied that the dream
on the imaginary screen cannot be further improved in any way,
have him or her take a step into the TV and be there just as though
really in the middle of the dream (an example of association into

the experience) and run it through again. Finally, give suggestions that he or she can do the same thing – i.e., change the ending
– while asleep and dreaming. You can include some direct suggestions for safety, strength and so forth, and explain that he or she is
now older, stronger, more informed, more prepared or safer, or in
some way more able to deal with the problem in a more appropriate way.

Summary: Disturbing Dreams and Nightmares

- Elicit the dream.

- Use a rewind procedure on the dream.

- Visualise and change the dream in some way; use cartoon
  imagery, change the ending, empower the child to do what is
  necessary.

- Direct suggestions for the child to realise he or she is dreaming
  and change the dream even while still asleep.

- Guided visualisation of child sleeping calmly all night long.

- Ego strengthening.

- Consider giving suggestions for sleeping on the right side (see
  research below).

- Suitable scripts: Choose extracts from any scripts in this chapter
  and also from Chapter 7 on anxiety.

An interesting small study, Agargu et al. (2004) was carried out
to discover whether different sleeping positions affected dream
characteristics, emotions and quality of sleep as subjectively experienced in men and women with no particular sleeping difficulties.
Forty-one slept on their right sides and 22 slept on their left sides.
Among the findings, the researchers discovered that the rate of
nightmare sufferers was reported as significantly higher in left-side
sleepers (40.9%) than in right-side sleepers (14.6%), with right-side
sleepers experiencing greater feelings of safety than their left-
side counterparts. Although these results are from a small study,
they suggest that dreaming and sleep quality may be affected by
sleep position, so it may be worth suggesting that children who

regularly report suffering from nightmares should try sleeping on their right sides. You will need to be clear in your suggestion that you are talking about the right side of the body not the bed!

Sleeping Script: Deal with unwanted night-time thoughts

Age range: approximately 9 years upward

I'm not going to suggest of course that you *sleep right now* ... only that you ... take some time to enjoy yourself ... as you daydream ... and all of the time that you ... *drift and dream* ... you can be aware that you have a thinking mind and a dreaming mind ... and when your thinking mind drifts off to some special place ... your dreaming mind knows how to ... *allow yourself to daydream* ... *daydream of something really special* ... so that's fine ... *go ahead and dream* ... dreaming of whatever lovely thing you like ... delightful even ... after all it's your mind, it's your dream ... and as you dream ... if any unwanted thought were to drift into your mind ... you could *imagine taking a large, white sheet of paper* ... and would you like a gold glitter pen? ... To *write down or draw any unwanted thought* that might just pop into your mind ... or would you prefer a paintbrush and paint box too? ... So you can *paint any old worry on to the paper* ... that's right ... *paint it right out of you.* ☺ **Pause for about half a minute or until you see that the child has stopped acting out the painting.** ☺ And when you've finished ... *fold the paper in half* ...and then in half again ... and keep folding it until it is so tiny ... you can *squeeze it into a matchbox* ... and put it in a drawer so it can *stay there all night through* ... *sleep there all night through* ... and you *put it right out of your mind* ... *put it completely out of your mind* ... you can *relax now* ... and every night while you sleep ... you can *sleep calmly and quietly all night through.*

And that's what you can do any night ... if ever any unwanted thought were to pop into your mind ... you can pop it into your matchbox and into your drawer so *that you forget all about it* ... or you could even imagine looking up into a blue sky with some fluffy clouds ... and let that thought float up and settle into a passing cloud ... and watch it *drift away* ... and as it drifts ... passing by the sun ... the rays of the sun burn through the cloud ... and burn away any old unwanted thought ... it just disappears.

Much better to think about these things in the daytime if you need to ... if you were even to bother to remember them ... you could take them out of your drawer and see that they *seem so much less important now* ... when you feel less drowsy than you *do feel drowsy right now* ... *too much effort to bother thinking now* ... and as you drift and dream now ... and feeling pleasantly drowsy ... I'm wondering if your arms are all floppy and tired? ... Do your arms feel heavier than your legs ... or do your legs feel heavier than your arms? ... Funny how when your hands begin to ... *relax more and more* that sometimes it almost seems … as if you *can't feel them at all* … it almost seems as if you can't feel your fingers at all.

And as you *rest … later at night … and every night* … you can *wait patiently for sleep* to slip over you like a soothing duvet … quietly and calmly … you *feel quiet and calm on the inside … feel quiet and calm* on the outside … inside out … quiet and calm … and as you *become ever more aware of the comfort spreading calm* … that ever growing feeling of calm comfort allows you to … *enjoy the rest* … all the way through … I wonder as you sit there so comfortably … how … at the same time you … see some kind of *picture* of yourself … chilling out … just there in your bed … enjoying the comfort … some people can *see* themselves … just loving the calm, inner comfort … other people just *feel* it on the inside … other people seem to *hear their inner voice soothing them* … reminding themselves of how calm and peaceful they feel … it seems so good to be in this place of effortless relaxation … and enjoying the drifting down and drifting up … and drifting away, not really wanting to make an effort … so just allowing it to happen … all on its own … every night … seems to be just the thing you want to do right now … and merely notice the drifting down … and drifting back … that's fine … drifting up and drifting down … drifting away to enjoy your dream … so that when you wake in the morning … you feel fantastic, full of energy … for while you are sleeping at night … your body is storing all of its energy for tomorrow … and as you relax now for a few moments more … I want you to know that *each day you become more and more calm and confident* … that *each night* … you *become more and more able to drift off* … into a *wonderful, quietly calm sleep* … you trust your special dreaming mind to look after you …to *keep you safe all night through* … so *every day, every night you expect to enjoy your rest … enjoy your sleep* … quietly… calm … happy … and, if you should half wake for a moment, or two … you will hear my words … quietly … calm … and immediately you will drift back to *sleep all night through.*

But for now of course it's not the time to sleep … it's the time to begin to drift back to the room with me. ☻ **Be sure to remove all suggestions for heaviness and sleep as you reorient the child to the room.** ☻

Sleeping Script: Whisper away night-time worries

Age range: approximately 5–8/9 years

So, right now you can take some time to enjoy yourself … and *have a little daydream* … right here in the chair … and as you daydream … your very special inside mind can find its own very special way to help you later when you're in bed … *have this very lovely daydream all over again* … all by yourself … well, with teddy/mousey/other favourite bedtime toy by your side of course …and all of the time that you … *dream* … you can *feel so happy* … so that's fine … go ahead and … can you see? Now … in your dream … you're in a magic garden … with the greenest, greenest grass you've ever seen … and the bluest, bluest sky ... and feel the gentle yellowy-orange, warm sun on your arms and legs ... and teddy can *feel the warmth too* ... and you and teddy can walk down the path ... and look at the bright, coloured flowers ... look at that lovely orange one over there ... it's calling out to you ... 'Hello ... I'm the magic worry flower ... I can help you if you've got any worries ... all you have to do is to pick me and tell me your worries ... and I will take them all away from you so you *can just relax and enjoy yourself.'*

Now doesn't that sound like a good idea? ... So why not pick the orange flower and *whisper your worries* into the petals/into the middle of it ... that's it ... brilliant ... and when you've finished ... let teddy have a go too ... tell him to *whisper anything that worries* him at all so the flower can take it ... and there's *no need to think about those things any more* ... great, now when you've completely finished ... both of you can *blow as hard as you can* at the petals and *blow them right away* ... and ... guess what ... as you blow those petals away ... those old thoughts get blown away too ... look ... maybe you can see them blowing right away in the wind ... and you can *feel so happy* ... and feel so relaxed ... and feel a bit sleepy ... look at teddy yawning ... *oh what a big yawn* ... has he already picked one of those sleepy, bluey coloured flowers just there? ... Because when you touch them ... they *make you yawn* ... that's right ... *just yawn like that* ... and when you pick one and hold it in your hand ... it just *makes you feel so sleepy* that *the harder you try to stay awake, the more you want to go to sleep* ... so *every night when you go to bed* ... *from now on* ... you will *drift off* to your magic garden ... *your dreams will always take you there* ... you and teddy ... and you can *pick a worry flower* if you want to ... and *tell it anything that upsets you* ... and *blow the petals and the worries away* ... and *feel so happy and comfy* ... sooo happy and comfy ... and then if you're still awake ... you can *pick the sleepy, bluey-coloured flower* ... that makes you yawn ... *really yawn* ... just like teddy ... *yawn your way to sleep.*

But right now of course it isn't really the time to go to sleep ... right now it's time to begin to wake up bright and happy ... wide, wide awake and happy that now you *know that every night* when you go to bed you will go to your special magic garden ... take teddy or whoever you want with you ... and find that *you are so comfy and sleepy that you yawn your way to sleep* ... and I wonder whether you will even have the time to pick your flowers because you *will be sooo tired and sleepy and happy and comfy* ... but of course right now it's the time to come back to the room with me ... feeling all your fingers and toes wanting to wriggle about ... feeling your whole body waking up and wanting to have a wonderful stretch right now.

Sleeping Script: Sounds don't bother you at all

Age range: approximately 8–12 years

I'd like you to begin by just allowing your eyelids to close … you can let all the tiny, tiny little muscles in your eyelids *relax* … can you believe there are hundreds … hundreds of tiny little muscles, nerve endings in your eyelids? … So don't worry about the *rest* of you … just allow your eyelids to *rest now* … so, the rest of you is ready to rest and my voice will help you to *relax and feel so comfy* as you go to bed and *rest and stay quietly calm all night through* … that's right… making them more comfortable now … really, *really let them relax* … and let the comfy feelings spread right through … *really feel them* … and as you *listen* to the sound of my voice … and as those *safe, comfy feelings grow* … you can just begin to *notice them spreading* … all over your body … all down through your tummy to the tips of your toes … and all over your mind … and every place that they touch in your mind and body … can *notice how comfy and dreamy you feel right now* … and it's alright … it's alright to let them feel more comfy all over, all the way through … and *it's safe to feel very, very comfy on the inside* … on the outside, inside out … *it's very safe to feel comfy and just listen to the sound of my voice* … really concentrating on the sound of my voice … so that … until I ask you to notice the sound of the clock/birds/your breathing/the traffic you were hardly aware of it at all … because those sounds (Child's Name) are not important to you at all … and now again … as you *really listen to my voice* … *hardly aware of the sounds in the room* … that's right … *hardly aware of the other sounds at all* … you know they are there, of course but … in a funny kind of a way … it's just as if *they're NOT there* … they're just in the background and you hardly take any notice of them and I want you to know that *from now on* … you can know the sounds are there at bedtime … the normal everyday sounds of the house … just sound normal to you … because of course they *are* normal … just like when they're there in the day-time and *you forget about them altogether* … you are so busy noticing different things … you're so busy daydreaming about your favourite game/your favourite doll/your PlayStation … from now on you will feel safe to know the sounds are there at night just as they are in the daytime and you hardly notice them at all.

And when I go to bed … I always like to (Child's Name) imagine that the radiators gurgling or the floorboards creaking … are the sounds of them having a conversation/a little chat as I *drift off to sleep* … and when you find that you can *think that too* … many of these normal, everyday, homely sounds can just *seem* to … *drift off into the distance* … so you … *hardly notice them at all … hardly notice them at all* … in fact, they can let you know that *everything is normal … everything is just as it should be* … and you can *drift off to sleep* knowing that everything is just normal … and it's normal for you to *feel comfy, calm and relaxed* as you drift and dream your way into *sleep*.

And isn't it funny how from now on (Child's Name) the sounds of the wind/the traffic/the television/the people talking and laughing can actually help you to *feel at ease* because you *know that this is how things should be … this is normal*

... in fact the very funny thing now is that ... *the more you try to listen to these sounds, the more tired you feel* ... and the more you try to listen, the more you listen to your own inner voice reminding you *everything is fine ... everything is normal* ... and you feel so sleepy that it's really hard to keep awake ... in fact ... *the harder you even try to stay awake, the sleepier you feel* ... the harder you were even to try to stay awake, the sleepier you feel.

So just before we finish, I'd like you to imagine yourself at home now in your bed ... see yourself there looking so comfy and sleepy ... how do you know you are so sleepy? ... Is it that your arms and legs are so floppy and tired? ... Are your eyelids really tired and heavy ... do you look really peaceful? ... Just drifting off to sleep ... and hear those old sounds of the wind/traffic/floorboards etc ... and notice how you say to yourself, 'Oh, it's just the wind/floorboards, etc., everything is fine ... everything is normal' and just *turn over and feel so sleepy and comfy that you just drift off to sleep* ... and just as you drift off to sleep ... you remember just how much mummy/daddy/granny/grandpa love you (Child's Name) ... and you feel so happy because you know they love you ... just because you're you ... *a really special person to be.*

But, of course, right now it's the time to come back to the room with me ... feeling all your fingers and toes wanting to wriggle about ... feeling your whole body waking up and wanting to have a wonderful stretch right now.

Suggestions for fear of the dark

You may incorporate one or more of these suggestions into a general sleeping script as you think appropriate to age, personality or the particular anxiety.

Triggered direct suggestion

As soon as you close your eyes ... you *think of your favourite place/magic garden/favourite activity* and you can *feel very comfy/safe/calm/relaxed ... you feel so relaxed that it doesn't seem to matter if it's light or dark because you feel very light and happy inside.*

Confusional reframe

Now you *stop* and *think about it in a new way*, you can *realise that the dark is always there* ... and *you're perfectly happy* ... it's just that the sun shines a light on it ... or *WE* switch the light on it ... the *darkness is always there underneath the light* and we *are perfectly safe* ... and when you think about it in this different way ... just as we are perfectly safe ... when the dark is all around UNDERNEATH the light ... we *can be perfectly safe* when the dark is all around ON TOP of the light ... you can *feel perfectly alright/happy/comfortable in the dark* ... and now you *really understand deep down and all the way through ... (the night)* ... how you can *feel so okay in the dark* ... you can *feel completely light-hearted/okay about being in the dark* in the evening and at

170

night … all the way through all right … all the way through the night … all the way through the night.

Guided visualisation

And now you *think differently* and you *feel differently* … have a look at that television and turn on the (Child's name) channel. Can you see (Child's name) in his/her bedroom? Look he/she's in bed and hey, what's different about him/her? You'll need to shine your torch on him/her to get a good look because it's quite dark. Brilliant! … He/she looks so comfy … how do you know he/she's comfy … does he/she look all floppy and tired? … And he/she looks so happy … how do you know he/she looks happy? … Does he/she have a little smile on his/her face? … And he/she looks so relaxed … and he/she feels so brave … and he/she feels so calm … and he/she feels so confident … and he/she looks so sleepy that maybe you want to take a big step into the television and be there now … and *really feel how comfy you are inside* … that's right … *feel so happy to know that you can sleep anywhere you like* … in the light … in the dark … *the dark doesn't bother you at all now … the dark doesn't bother you at all* … in fact … you *hardly bother to notice the dark at all* except to know that when *it's nice and dark you can go to sleep really easily … sleep really quickly indeed.*

Ideas for very young ones

Take them off to fairyland and have the magic fairy/wizard look after them all night long. Get the fairy or wizard to sprinkle magic light dust into the dark so they can feel just as happy in the dark as in the light.

Chapter Eleven

Being Bullied

Bullying and Possible Effects

The following are common forms of bullying but the list is by no means exhaustive.

Verbal

This type of bullying includes: direct name-calling; talking behind a child's back; insulting his or her family; continual teasing about appearance, lack of wealth or any perceived weak point; and racial slurs or sexual harassment. These attacks can be in person or through text messaging, phone calls, emails and graffiti.

Emotional

Emotional bullying can include: deliberately leaving someone out of the conversation, game or other activity; stealing, hiding, or damaging his or her possessions; threatening and humiliating the person, and then taunting him or her for blushing or crying in response.

Physical

Physical bullying covers a broad range of contact: pinching, pushing, restraining, spitting, kicking, hitting, forcing a person to give up money or possessions, sexual touching or threats of unwanted physical advances, and any violent or intimidating behaviour.

It is commonly stated in school policies that for behaviour to be defined as bullying, it must be intentional and repeated. The fact is, however, that if a child feels bullied, the effect is the same whether the bully planned the attack or acted on impulse and engaged in what he or she claimed was merely some 'mild teasing'.

Possible Effects on the Child

- low self-esteem, anxiety, fear, depression.

- embarrassment, shame, becoming withdrawn and shy of social contact.

- difficulty in sleeping and fatigue.

- underachievement at school, school phobia.

- loss of interest in hobbies.

- self-harming behaviour, or even threatened, attempted or actual suicide.

Bullying is carried out in a variety of everyday situations and can sometimes be perpetrated by children, adults, families, strangers, so-called 'friends' and, sadly, even teachers. It commonly occurs on the way to and from school and in the playground.

Bullying is a serious problem and children need to be encouraged to confide in their parents and teachers for support. They should not be expected to deal with it on their own. All schools should have an active bullying policy in place and if a case is not being dealt with effectively, there are procedures for parents to follow. (Go to www.Kidscape.org.uk for helpful resources.)

Suitable Aims for Hypnotherapy Treatment

What Can Be Achieved With Hypnotherapy?

Check that the aims of parents and children are realistic (see the list that follows) and that they understand that hypnotherapy in itself will not stop the bullying. If the bullying is relatively mild and the child feels able to be assertive, it *may* result in the bullying stopping or reducing but if bullying has gone a stage further than this, clearly other measures need to be taken as well. Usually this next step will involve parents and schools playing an important part and I believe that, as therapists, we need to guard against falling into the trap of becoming over involved and thinking that we should have the answer to every problem that comes our way. The website and books recommended in the useful resources section are extremely helpful for parents, children and hypnotherapists.

I have had more than one father whose expectations have been that I should hypnotise their rather gentle, frightened boy into being able to stand up to a whole group of bullies and literally fight them all. Clearly, this is not the answer to the problem, and it may in fact cause the child to feel under even more pressure. It could also result in a real threat to the child's safety. However, the hypnotic visualisation of the child seeing him or herself using appropriate assertiveness skills rather than aggression should certainly go some way towards helping the child out of victim thinking.

Specific Goals

- Give an opportunity to relax and release tension.

- Raise self-esteem and confidence level.

- Help children realise that it is not their fault and they do not deserve to be bullied.

- Help them cope with their own emotions more resourcefully.

- Help them find strategies to emotionally dissociate from name calling or verbal abuse.

- Teach some simple body language that is more positive and assertive.

- Help them to understand that a positive thought on the inside can cause a positive effect on their facial expression and body language.

- Teach strategies that are more assertive (not aggressive) and get them to visualise themselves carrying them out.

The aims should be 100% negotiated with and agreed upon by the child, the parent and the therapist to ensure that neither the parent nor the therapist can in any way be in danger of imposing inappropriate ideas that could backfire and make the situation worse than it already is. Enormous care should be taken not to encourage children to put themselves in physical danger. If in any doubt, err on the side of caution and always include ego strengthening in addition to any other chosen intervention.

The Use of Anchors

A very useful technique to help a child deal with bullying is to install an anchor (or trigger) for confidence and resourcefulness. The process is explained in Chapter 7, and the script 'Treasure hunt' can be adapted for use in situations in which children are being bullied. The technique makes use of anchors to help remain calm, confident and in control in any situation.

Scripts for Different Ages

Inductions

The choice of a simple, progressive relaxation induction would be appropriate for an initial treatment when the primary aims may be relaxation, release of anxiety and ego strengthening. As the child breathes out, have him or her breathe out any old, unwanted stored anxieties on the out breath and breathe in calm and comfort with every in breath.

At a subsequent session the use of a finger or hand levitation induction (see Chapter 2) may serve as a powerful argument for the power of the unconscious mind. Giving back a sense of inner control to a child who is being bullied is of paramount importance. However, bear in mind that the child usually needs to be of a certain level of maturity to understand fully that movements may be driven at the unconscious level. The effect is not the same when a child consciously moves his or her hand in order to please the therapist. A suggestion that tingling should be experienced in the fingers can be substituted for lifting; it is effective and normally well accepted.

The following script/conversation, 'Shrink the bully', helps a child to feel more resourceful. Not only can bullying cause physical or emotional pain at the time it takes place, but also the effects can linger and cause anxiety and lowered self-esteem that lasts throughout childhood and beyond. By changing children's attitudes and helping them to feel even a little more empowered and resourceful, you can help to limit the damage. Children usually enjoy the following suggestions because they give them a sense of being in control, help counter 'victim' thinking and introduce an element of humour into an otherwise miserable situation. I frequently use this activity while chatting and then again later as reinforcement in a more formal trance state. You can teach it as a tool to be used to counter anxious thoughts when children are on their own. The questions within the script are genuine rather than rhetorical. Make a note of their answers as you go along.

The rationale for first making the mental image of the bully bigger and more frightening is twofold:

- You can check that the size and proximity of the image the child sees in his or her mind's eye are important factors in making the bully appear more frightening and overpowering. If so, and they usually are, you know that these are the aspects that you need to manipulate, making them smaller and more distant.

- You utilise the child's fear response. Initially the child may resist shrinking down an imaginary image of the bully because the fear is too strong; so you do the unexpected and encourage him or her to make it bigger (and probably more frightening) which is easy for them to do. Paradoxically, the fact that they *can increase* the size of their mental picture means that they have actually exerted some mental control and are thus more able to *decrease* the size as a subsequent step. This naturally results in the sought-after lessening of anxiety.

Interactive Script: Shrink the bully

Age range: approximately 6 years upward

(Note that masculine pronouns are being used in this script, but that the feminine should be used if appropriate.)

Close your eyes and imagine the person/the bully standing in front of you.

What does he look like? … Now make him look bigger and closer. Does that make him look better or worse? … ☜ **Likely to make the image more disturbing.** ☜

Okay. Now make him smaller and move him right away from you. Good … put him right over there by the door. How does he look/seem now? … ☜ **Likely to make the image less disturbing.** ☜ Brilliant … now I want you to shrink him down smaller and smaller … just like in the film 'Honey, I Shrunk the Kids'! That's it. Shrink him right down … cut him right down to size so you can pick him up in your hand and squash him even smaller … great. Now get him so, so tiny that you can pop him into that matchbox/drawer/jam jar … how does that feel? Feel good? … Great, from now on I want you to know that whenever you have a thought that used to worry you about any silly, unkind person who has been trying to bully you in any way … you will automatically be able to shrink him down in your mind and … as you capture him in your matchbox … you can *put him right out of your mind* so the thought of him *won't bother you at all … no longer upsets you in any way* … you will just understand that he is a very small-minded person and you won't even bother to waste your time thinking about him at all … in fact the harder you try to remember to think about him … the more you seem to *forget about him.*

Bullying Script: Protective bubble (for children subjected to verbal taunting or abuse)

Age range: approximately 8–12 years

I want you to know that the very special part of you that knows how to look after you has been listening harder and harder and has been coming up with a plan to help you *deal with these boys/girls/bullies/the situation in a much more confident way,* a plan to help you find that *the silly/unkind/unpleasant things they say seem to wash right over you … as of no importance at all.*

And you can already begin to see part of the plan … as you look in your mind's eye and notice that just above you there is a bubble, which is very flexible/bendy and you can pull it into any shape that you want … just do that now … pull it and stretch it and see that it can form any shape you want … that's right … this is your *protective* bubble, a bit like bubble wrap but so much stronger … and you can *pull that bubble down over you* so it's protecting you from anything, any silly names on the outside, so that you feel perfectly okay on the inside. … notice how the colour has become completely transparent so you can see right through it … nobody else can *see that bubble* except you because *it's your very own protective bubble* … so anybody who calls you names can't *see them bouncing off* … but *you* can *see the names bounce off* … that's right … listen, can you hear them? What sort of sound do they make as they bounce right off? ☞ **If you are clever at such things, you might want to put in some appropriate sound effects here; otherwise, the child can just imagine the sounds.** ☜ It doesn't matter what they say now … the words just bounce right off, don't they? … You are strong … you are so much more confident now … s*ee them, hear them …* maybe you can even *feel them bouncing off* as you *stay calm and confident* on the inside, protected by your very own invisible bubble … you know that nothing they say can upset you or worry you in that same old way ever again … you are strong and brave and confident and you just look the other way and walk on.

☞ **At this point, you can personalise the suggestions to the individual situation. Get the child to watch a mental film in which he or she is able to cope coolly and calmly, being powerfully aware of the invisible protection, which nobody else can see.** ☜

Brilliant! See how much more confident you look … look at the expression on your face … you've actually got a smile on your face … look at you walking to school/in the playground, etc. … you're ignoring those silly children because *you know that now, with your invisible bubble/coat/shield of protection, whatever they say means nothing to you.*

Who will be most surprised that *you are calm and in charge/in control of your feelings*? Who will be most pleased that *you can ignore them now*? Will it be your mum/dad/teacher etc. when you tell them? … Or will it be *you who is most pleased and proud of yourself*? … Maybe the bullies themselves will be surprised and a bit disappointed that *you have stopped reacting when they tease you* … and I want you to know that your very special … inner mind will be sorting out the rest of the plan each night as you sleep so that it finds a way for you to *stay in control of your feelings* without even noticing you're doing it … and each day you feel stronger and stronger … more and more confident … more and more positive … and more and more determined to enjoy being you … an exceptionally nice person to be.

179

☞ When you bring the child back, remember to remove suggestions for lightness and have him or her take off the protective shield, bubble, coat, etc., and keep it in his or her pocket, ready to take out whenever it is needed. You may also want to give suggestions for the child to report the behaviour, but only do this if it has previously been negotiated with both the child and parent. ☜

Bullying Script: Museum of your mind (Building confidence, resilience and positive thinking)

Age range: approximately 10/12 years upward

And feeling more comfortable, feeling more relaxed ... and to make you *feel even more comfortable* ... I wonder if you can *use your imagination right now* ... and imagine that the air around you is a wonderful colour that reminds you of every positive and confident feeling or thought you've ever had ... I wonder what colour that would be? ... And with each breath you take ... *see it filling your body ... feel it balancing your body and mind ... hear it filling your mind with positive and confident thoughts and feelings* ... that's right ... the colour spreading all around now as you begin to *remember some of those positive happy times in your life right now.*

Now look a little more closely ... can you notice any other areas that have a different colour? ... The colour of any possible tension or anxiety or low feeling perhaps? ... I wonder what colours those would be. ... Well, have a look and if there are any, begin to *breathe those colours out of your body* ... right out of your mind ... *breathe out that tension ... breathe out those anxious feelings ... breathe out any sad thoughts* ... and *breathe in that wonderful colour of calm, confident feelings* ... and let it *spread all around your body and mind* ... that's right, that's brilliant ... you can do this whenever you want to *feel rather more calm and confident.*

And in this comfortable slightly dreamy state you have become very imaginative and creative ... I want to talk to you about the museum of your mind which has been collecting positive experiences ever since the day you were born ... there are many different rooms with different collections ... one stores all our memories, stores our feelings and beliefs about ourselves and our abilities and stores our habits too ... another collects our best exhibits ... a bit like a gallery of all our achievements ... there's a reference section too that stores information and knowledge ... there are curators who guard the collections and decide what is valuable and what is to be stored and what is not ... I'd like you to take a walk around your different collections ... let's go first to the gallery of achievements ... *your very own* achievements ... things that you are good at, things that you enjoy, things you've done ... sometimes it's an achievement that other people know about and sometimes it's just one that you know yourself ... it could be something that you wrote or even thought, could be a match you won, a goal you scored ... or was it when you first learned to ride a bike, or played some sport, or sang or danced, or played and listened to music that you love? ... Was it when you designed or constructed something and were really proud of what you'd done? ... Was it when you suddenly understood something that had been a bit difficult for you or you mastered a computer game? ... Or maybe you helped a friend, or you were especially thoughtful and loving to friends and family? ... Maybe *you are brilliant* about being kind and getting on with people ... all of these things are very valuable indeed ... just as *YOU are very valuable indeed* ... so just walk around in here and *enjoy looking at the exhibits ...* they may even sometimes be hidden in a corner under a cover because it's been a long time since you came in here and had a good look around. ... hey, look over there on the wall, there's a certificate ... it's got your name on it ... It says you've been awarded this certificate for coping really well with challenging situations. ☜ **Insert something you have elicited in your pre-trance talk, or point out that the child has done well in having coped thus far even though the bullying made him or her unhappy.** ☜ Well done ... that's a very useful quality to have. It helps you *cope with all kinds of things in your life ...* Look over there at the curator sitting on that chair by the door ... does he look wide awake or could he be having a little doze? ... It's very important that he does his job properly. ... first of all he should be going around the collection to uncover achievements that may have got hidden behind something or need a polish ... if you need to, go and wake him up and show him how to *look in every nook and cranny* ... every little corner so you can *discover positive qualities and achievements* that have been forgotten over time ... do that now. ☜ **Long pause.** ☜ Good.

And there's another very important part of the curator's job too ... it's to check that nobody sneaks anything into the room that really shouldn't be there ... if he's dozing, stuff can get stored in there that isn't helpful ... maybe unhelpful negative opinions or beliefs about ourselves which can stop us being the strong confident people we really are meant to be ... (we really are meant to *be confident*).

Sometimes there are bullies who like to call people names ... try to put us down for some reason ... or maybe they are jealous of us ... or sometimes even, *they* feel better through trying to make someone else feel bad (how strange is that?) ... And then sometimes that negative stuff gets sneaked into our own collection when no one is paying attention ... maybe you've stored some rubbish too? ... Perhaps something that was even meant to be a silly joke ... sometimes you could even have misunderstood what they meant. ... some stupid name or untrue label but you let it hurt you at the time ... could have come from anywhere, a child, someone you know or someone you hardly know, a so-called friend, possibly even a teacher, but for whatever reason they had the wrong idea about you.

I want you to know that those messages are very mistaken and not to be accepted or believed at all ... so I want you to have a walk around all the rooms in the museum ... especially the ones that store your beliefs and opinions about yourself ... go in now and find any stupid name, or mistaken belief or unhelpful opinion that really belonged to somebody else but for whatever reason you took it in and made it your own … and you let it grow and develop so it became even more upsetting … or even worse … perhaps you began to believe it too! … Isn't that strange?

Believe me, these are very mistaken and extremely damaging and certainly have no place in your museum … so when you find one, I want you immediately to *turf/chuck it out of that room* … get the curator to help you if it's a bit heavy … and *chuck it out* into the rubbish bin/the trash can where it belongs with all the other trash … It doesn't belong to you and it had no business being there in the first place! … What's more, you need to get rid of any negative, sad or under-confident feeling connected with it too … that's really important … great … take your time and get rid of all the trash … and nod your head when you've finished. ☜ **Pause and observe carefully. You will often see movements in the hands, body and or eyes as the child engages in this activity.** ☞

Good, excellent! Wasn't that satisfying! … Of course the important thing now is to make sure that you have worthwhile thoughts and feelings in your gallery … take all the time you need now to paint a fantastic picture or form/mould a wonderful sculpture that is full of bright, strong confident feelings … make sure it has strong positive statements and beliefs that will grow stronger and stronger as you get into the habit of … thinking positively about yourself … *think positively about yourself* … so as you paint, or mould the sculpture, you will hear me give you some very positive messages that you will incorporate into/include in your very own masterpiece/work of art. ☜ **Use your judgment as to whether to use 'I' or 'You' in the following affirmations.** ☞

- I am bright and I can learn to program positive thoughts very well/use positive thinking.

- I already have many strengths and from now on I will remember these strengths.

(Go on … let your memory remind you again of something you do really well or some positive quality you have).

- I can learn to be more confident in my ability to dismiss negative thoughts and think positive thoughts each day.

Good. Well Done. Keep painting or sculpting.

- I can dismiss negative thoughts whenever I want to.

- If anybody dares to sneak in any stupid name or harmful message, my curator will notice it and wash it off immediately … he's on the alert now.

- Everyday I am becoming stronger and stronger in my mind.

- I can shrug off remarks and refuse to let them get to me/upset me.

- Great. Now you've got the idea, why don't you include a couple of positive messages of your own? And nod your head when you've done it. ☺ **Long pause.** ☺

Good, very well done indeed … so just before we finish I would like you to move into the interactive section in the museum … sit in the chair in front of the screen where you can see into the future … zoom forward into a few weeks from now where you will have got rid of any negative exhibits and find that you have absorbed the positive beliefs from your new pictures and sculptures … hey, *look at you in and around school, so self-assured and calm! You look so much more upbeat and smiling* … listen to your voice as *you are even able to turn something into a joke* when anybody tries to make fun of you … well done … notice how surprised those people are that you are no longer looking sad or upset by them … you know your own value … you are very valuable indeed.

Now have a look at you when you're at home and notice how *you are refusing to dwell on negative thoughts* … and, as it is becoming second nature to you to *stop negative thoughts* as soon as they begin, *you are focusing on something positive* and enjoying your memory reminding you of all those great qualities you have … you are visiting the wonderful new collections in the museum of your mind and you are feeling amazing!

And in a moment I'm going to count from 1 to 10 and bring you back from the museum and … as I count upward you will feel all the energy coming back into your body … any tired heavy feelings will be removed … and by the time I reach the number 8, your eyelids will feel light and want to open wide … and by the time I reach the number 10, you will be back here with me feeling bright and positive and so much more optimistic/positive than you've felt in a long, long time.

I want you to know that as the days and the weeks and the months go by you will become ever stronger and more resourceful … you will find it easier and easier to *refuse to let stupid remarks affect you* in any way except to *make you stronger and more resilient* … you will *remain calm and confident* and able to *deal with things in an easier, more carefree way* … as you *get emotionally stronger* all the time, your body language will naturally become more confident and easy within yourself and you will *become more at ease with those around you.*

Remember you are a valuable person … *a*nd I wonder whether you will surprise yourself or whether it will seem perfectly normal that you are finding so many new ways to *practise respecting yourself every day* … and you know, you don't even have to *focus very closely on your own positive qualities and abilities* because now your memory will remind you of them more and more each day.

Bullying Script: Defeat the bully

Age range: approximately 8 years upward (depending on how you choose to adapt specific vocabulary and ideas)

This script is slightly complex and needs reading carefully before use, but it will appeal to a child who is visual and is familiar with interactive computer games.

> ☜ **You need to make it clear in your pre-trance discussion with the child that you are not suggesting that he or she does or says anything that will provoke physical violence, only that the child thinks and acts in a more confident way, maybe making use of distraction or humour. ☜**

And sitting here so comfortably, I'd like you to imagine that you are sitting in front of your computer/PlayStation and you are going to play the game, 'Defeat the Bully' ... so switch everything on and get settled down ... nod your head when you are ready to start ... great.

Now the first thing to remember is that there are different ways to defeat a bully. But before we can do that we have to think about how bullies win their nasty games. How do they know they have won? Well, one way is that they get the reaction from you that they want ... so, what do they want? ... Maybe they want to make you feel sad or angry or upset or maybe they want to make you cry, and in some peculiar way, then they can feel better about themselves. How pathetic is that! ... And the way they are going to know that they have won is to see you display/show those feelings.

One way you can learn to defeat the bully is to become a very good actor and *act as though you feel perfectly fine* thank you very much! ... And an even better way than acting as though *you are perfectly fine* ... is to *feel perfectly fine* without even acting at all! ... Now here's the thing ... maybe you FIRST have to learn how to *think in a positive way* and ACT *perfectly fine on the outside* and THEN, with practice, the *perfectly fine feelings will come along all by themselves* and you will *feel perfectly fine inside* ... and as you *learn to do this more and more easily*, you will know that *you are the winner.*

Now, look at the game on the screen and see those children over there ... pick out the ones who look happy and confident and then pick out the ones who are a bit sad and a bit anxious and not very confident ... good ... how do you know which ones are which? ... Can you see that the ones who are happy and confident are more relaxed in their bodies but they are naturally standing up straighter? ... Do they somehow look more bouncy? ... Do their faces look more smiley? ... Do they look as if they have more energy and are thinking positive and happy thoughts? ... You're quite right ... now look at the kid with the most worried/miserable expression or downbeat body language ... do you think this kid looks as if he has a positive opinion about himself? ... Do you think he's thinking 'I'm happy and I'm intelligent/smart' or something more like 'I'm really fed up' or 'I'm a bit stupid'? ... Okay, you're right. He's probably NOT thinking 'I'm happy' or 'I'm intelligent/smart' … here's the thing … when we *feel good inside* and when we *have a positive opinion* of ourselves, it shows in our face and it shows in our body … and when it shows in our face and it shows in our body we are less likely to be picked on.

So this is where you really start the game to defeat the bully. … I want you to imagine you have the control/mouse in your hand and in a moment you're going to click on a character to change the way he looks … but the way you're going to change the way this character looks on the outside is by changing the way he feels on the inside. … and you can change the way he feels on the inside by getting him *to think something positive* … so, look at the screen … look, there's a bully coming along and he's trying to decide which of the children in the group he wants to torment … he's going for the kid who looks least happy and least confident … Okay. Nod your head when you've found the kid who looks least happy and least confident … to score a point you have to help him change his expression by thinking really positively … click on him and give him a positive thought about himself … maybe you can tell him to remember something brilliant he's done … or something nice his mum/dad/granddad/best friend/etc. has said about him … or think about stroking a pet.

☞ Or you can insert something positive here that you have previously elicited from the child in your pre-trance chat. ☜

Has his expression changed yet? … If you need to make him look even more sure of himself, click on him and give him another positive thought … keep giving him more positive thoughts until his expression looks confident … right, now it's time to change his body language, so click on him and remind him about something that really made him laugh one day … and as he does, notice how his body language is changing to positive and bouncy … so he looks happy and more confident … and altogether more able to *deal more confidently with that bully when he starts his stupid teasing/taunting/name calling. …* nod your head when you've done it … as you look, notice how, now that he feels better about himself, that boy refuses to let the bully know he's upset even when the bully says something really nasty, or calls out a horrid name … he still keeps a confident look on his face … and also notice that the silly bully doesn't look quite so satisfied now that he hasn't quite got the reaction he wanted … so, great … you score another point … you are doing really well … you really *are* helping to defeat the bully!

Right, so now you've got the idea, you need to score some more points because the bully isn't giving up just yet. He's going to try again. … prepare your character so he can *feel strong and resourceful/full of good ideas. Click on him and tell him what to think …* 'I am strong. I can beat the bully. I'm going to think something really positive right now' … good … well done … now, this time when he hears the bully's voice, I want you to let him hear that voice in a squeaky Mickey Mouse voice so he sounds very silly indeed. He sounds so very silly when he says something that's meant to be nasty that it almost makes *you want to smile inside …* so when you can hear it in that silly, squeaky Mickey

Mouse voice and almost *smile inside* … I want you to click on your character, get him to look the bully in the eye and say something that will really surprise him because it has nothing to do with what he just said … something like … 'Hey, your trainers/jeans/hair cut look cool. Where did you get them?/Where did you have it done?'

☺ **You may also suggest that the child tell a silly one-line joke that has been practised in advance, or ask a question that doesn't have an easy answer. A little research in a trivia book will yield some fun facts: 'Do you know why snot is green'? (Because it's got bacteria in it.) 'Do you know why bird poo is white not black?' (It's not poo; it's pee!) Apparently, according to Mick O'Hare (2006), what we think is white poo is not really poo at all, it is urine.** ☺

What did the bully's face look like? … Did he look surprised? … A bit shocked perhaps? … Did your character keep his cool and *act as if he really is confident?* … Good … sounds as though you've scored another point … just click on him and try it again. The more often you do this, the better you get at it … maybe think of a different thing to say this time. ☺ **The next section of the script works best when you have already carried out the 'Shrink the bully' activity above.** ☺ Okay. Time to shrink the bully down to size … click on your character and tell him to look at that bully and imagine *he can shrink him right down and then put him in a matchbox* … that's right … another point … you really are getting very good at this … somehow when you can play about with him in your mind you feel so much more confident and so much more in control/in charge of your feelings.

☺ **Leave out the following short section about making a joke if the child is too young/too depressed/not creative enough to be able to do this successfully. If you decide to include it, any idea would certainly need to be discussed beforehand to ensure that it doesn't backfire and further damage the child's self-esteem. It can be a very positive strategy when it works (we know that most of the best comedians learned their skill in response to bullying), but it could be counterproductive if the task is just too difficult to manage.** ☺

On we go …

Let's think about another thing you could do to help defeat the bully … now *you're becoming a bit more confident,* could you … *have your character make a bit of a joke out of something,* perhaps? … Like, if the bully calls him 'fat face' or 'spotty' could he say, 'You haven't seen anything yet. I'm working on getting even fatter/spottier!' or 'I'm going to buy a Dalmatian/spotty dog to match' … the trick here is to make a joke on yourself *not on the bully*; that way the bully is more likely to laugh and secretly be a bit impressed … maybe you could even think about what you could say to YOUR bully and when you've come up with an idea, click on your character and get him to say it so it gets a laugh … (This is something you might really want to practise at home as well) … you get triple points if the bully laughs … 10 points if YOU laugh … and, even if nobody laughs, you get 5 points just for trying … nod your head when you're ready to move on. ☺ **Pause for a while and, if there is no nod of the head, ask if the child wants more time or wants to move on.** ☺

Good, you've done so well I'd like you to move on to the next level and click on the new game … and notice that the character on the screen is you in your very own situation … and I want you to do all the same kinds of things that you did before but this time click on yourself to make all the changes you need to … *stay calm and in charge of your own thoughts and feelings … talk to yourself in a very positive way … check that your body language looks confident* as you just listen to the sound of my voice relaxing you … each time you make a change in your thoughts or your expression or your body language I want you to nod your head and let me know.

☺ **Allow your patient the time to go through this in his or her head while you make very quiet relaxing and ego-strengthening suggestions in the background.** ☺

Brilliant, amazing! … And, feeling so strong and so much more resourceful/confident … I want you to know that nothing and nobody can worry or upset you in exactly that same old way … because you have found a way to *change the way you see things … change the way you think about things and change the way you feel about things on the inside …* now I'm not saying that that silly/pathetic person might not try again, as he may … but I *am* saying that as the days and the weeks and the months go by, you are becoming stronger and stronger … more and more able to deal with him in a different way … so you can *shrug him off and ignore him … get on with your life in a strong and confident way …* I want you to know that you've been amazing today and *the more often you do this in your mind the better you get at it. You are absolutely brilliant!*

Bullying Script: Cyber bullying

Age range: approximately 12 years upward

This script uses a framework of relaxing, comforting and strength building. There is a selection of practical suggestions included, which you can insert as suited to the individual situation. These need to be discussed and agreed upon beforehand, preferably with the parents involved since they may need to give practical assistance in changing phone numbers, blocking mails and reporting problems, etc. I suggest using a simple relaxing induction coupled with a favourite safe place since the child normally feels exhausted from the stress of being a target of cyber bullying. Add extra ego strengthening, perhaps selecting a script from Chapter 3.

As you sit there relaxing and enjoying the comfort of the chair … you can let my voice *comfort and relax you* more and more with each word you hear … *feel my voice comforting and relaxing you* … as you *go deeper and deeper relaxed* with each breath you take … CALM and RELAX … just listening and relaxing and accepting comforting words and *comfortable feelings increasing* … just listening and relaxing and *accepting the positive suggestions* which will improve your mood remarkably … CONFIDENT and STRONG … just listening and relaxing and accepting that these ideas will help you *cope more calmly* with everything that is happening around you … and as you *go deeper and deeper relaxed* and that *feeling of comfort grows inside* … and *spreads all through your mind and body* … I want you to know that your very special inner mind/unconscious mind is going to *help you today* find a way to *protect you every day* … STAY CONFIDENT and STRONG … protect you on the inside so that no matter how hard those bullies/unkind people/pathetic people try to hurt you … *you will stay strong and calm on the inside* … you refuse to let them get to you whatever they say … whatever they do … whatever messages they send … they may get to your phone but *they cannot get to you.*

And while your conscious mind can *drift and dream* when it wants to … I am going to ask your unconscious mind, which has steadily been becoming more and more attentive, to … *listen very carefully now* and use its very special power to protect the inner you … feel it happening now … CONFIDENT and STRONG … some people feel as if the inside self, which stores all your thoughts and feelings, is being shielded by some very strong protective perspex/toughened glass screen so that nothing and no one can dent your confidence … CONFIDENT and STRONG … no spiteful words and no untrue rumours can upset you … you know you have done nothing wrong … you do not deserve this treatment … as you listen to my voice now … your unconscious mind will remind you that the people who *really* know you well … your mum and dad (all relevant people) … *know you are a good/kind/thoughtful/intelligent/sensible person who deserves to be respected* … and as you listen now and you *feel calm and relaxed* … your inner confidence is growing stronger and stronger.

And feeling pleasantly aware now of how calm and relaxed you feel, I want to remind you of the best ways to help yourself get through these times in the best possible way for you.

℅ Select whatever is appropriate from this advice, having already discussed it in the pre-trance talk with both the child and parent. ℅

• Spend more time with people who you like and trust and who like and trust you.

• Always tell your family/your teacher/a very good friend what is happening … they can help you report it, if necessary … they can help you find out how to block messages from anybody who is behaving badly.

• Every time you block a message or a sender you get a surge of confidence.

- You will block the message from your mind so that it has no importance to you.

- Refuse to retaliate or reply to texts, emails or other messages … it would only encourage them and make things worse … you can rise above it and stay cool and in control.

- Don't put yourself in the wrong by sending a bad message back. Stay in the right. Remember that anything you send in anger can stay online and be used against you.

- Think before you speak and think before you send.

- If you really need to read a message to save the evidence, imagine your protective screen in front of the phone/computer so the words don't get to you … you are strong and protected and the words seem to have no meaning to you … they no longer upset you in that old way for you are strong and confident inside.

- Resist re-reading bullying texts that you have saved as evidence.

- Stay away from chat rooms/messaging services … every time you are tempted and you *resist that temptation to go there,* you *get a surge of confidence and respect for yourself.*

- Ask your family to help you change your phone number and then refuse to give it to anybody except your family and really trusted best friends.

- Keep any passwords a secret.

- **NB Only use the following suggestion if collection of evidence is not an issue:** Every time you delete a message or an email without looking at it, you get a surge of confidence.

Great … every night when you go to bed you can notice your breathing and use it to calm and strengthen you … begin to breathe away any uncomfortable thought or feeling on your out *breath* … mentally say the words CALM and RELAX … on your in *breath* … mentally see your perspex/toughened glass protection and say the words CONFIDENT AND STRONG and every day you become tougher and stronger so those messages no longer upset you in any way … you cope with anyone, anything and any situation in a strong and confident way.

Chapter Twelve

Behaviour Problems

Who is Likely to Present for Hypnotherapy Treatment?

- Children who have a diagnosis of Attention Deficit Hyper-activity Disorder (ADHD).

- Children who have a diagnosis of Oppositional Defiant Disorder (ODD).

- Children who display several of the symptoms but do not fulfil all the criteria for a diagnosis of ADHD or a diagnosis of ODD.

- Children who display typical 'naughty' childhood behaviours characteristic of most children at some stage in their development. Some or all of these behaviours will have become more frequent or more disruptive than previously. It may be that their behaviour has temporarily worsened because of changes in their school or home environment, for example bullying, new teacher, new class, peer pressure, new baby or marital disharmony. Reasons can be many and various and sometimes the parents' own inconsistent parenting style will impact negatively on their child's behaviour. It may be that in the very early years children were allowed to 'get away with' behaviour that has become less acceptable as they have grown older. It may be that parents are worn down through having been called in once too often to speak to school representatives about their child's behaviour. Children's behaviour can also vary considerably from home to school; they may be helpful and thoughtful in one environment and disruptive in the other.

What Types of Behaviour are Appropriate for Hypnotherapy Treatment?

Hyperactivity behaviours associated with the hyperactivity part of Attention Deficit Hyperactivity Disorder will often be quite responsive to hypnotherapy.

Children suffering from ADHD may tend to be:

*   Impulsive/restless/fidgety/excessively energetic/irritable/ argumentative/aggressive/disruptive/emotionally immature. They frequently have little or no fear of danger and ignore warnings, showing little awareness of consequences.

(The attention deficit behaviours of ADHD/ADD are discussed in Chapter 13.)

Children with Oppositional Defiant Disorder may tend to be:

*   quick to lose their temper/argumentative/non-compliant to adults' rules or requests/deliberately annoying to others/ blaming of others for their own misbehaviour/touchy, easily irritated or angered/resentful/spiteful/vindictive.

Of course, much of the above behaviour is just part and parcel of being a child and not symptomatic of any kind of disorder. However, when such behaviour causes real problems within the family or at school, it is certainly worth using hypnotherapy to help to manage it. When the child has already been diagnosed with one of the conditions mentioned, you can work with other health or educational professionals to support their behaviour management plans. As always, we aim to help *manage* rather than cure symptoms and we need to make this very clear to parents who may have different expectations.

The Essential Starting Point

Remember that we can never make any patient, child or adult, do something that he or she doesn't want to do, so it is absolutely crucial to find out whether or not the child wants to change the behaviour – and why. Getting the child on your side is essential, otherwise frustration and stalemate are what lie ahead. With this in mind, it is important to gather some case history information before seeing the child and parent together since it is decidedly unhelpful for the first session to consist merely of a long list of the child's misdeeds. This is not to suggest that problems should not be discussed honestly with the child present, but simply that there should be a concentration initially on the more important behavioural changes needed and that the discussion should be as free from recrimination as possible. Look back to Chapter 1 for general ideas within the solution-focused approach, which I have found immensely helpful when dealing with behaviour problems. Using these ideas I have normally been able to help children find reasons to want to make changes for themselves, even if it is, at first, only to get parents or teachers 'off their back'. Do not be put off by such a response, as it can be a reasonable motivation to work with and one that it is genuinely meaningful to the child. Other motivations may well follow; in fact, they usually do!

Just as you need to get the cooperation of the child, you need to get the cooperation of the parents and this will probably mean asking them to refrain from reminding the child about past misdemeanours and instead noticing, and giving them credit for, changes in current behaviour. It is also useful to remind them to be on the lookout for a lack of bad behaviour – perhaps an absence of sulkiness or cheeky responses – since these things often go unacknowledged but are actually very positive signs of progress indeed.

Explanations, Questions and Interventions

Notice that the words in italics form embedded commands, which are very effective when used during the information-gathering part of the conversation and during the trance state.

I'm a hypnotherapist, and my job is to help people get over their problems by using their minds/imaginations in a very special way. I've helped a lot of children around your age to get over this kind of problem/deal with temper problems. I've heard from your mum and dad that there have been some problems at school/at home/with losing your temper/with upsetting other children, so I've got a pretty good idea of why *they* would like me to help you but what I really need to know is why *you* would like me to help you. Is it actually true that *you* would like me to help you? What's in it for you?

So, are you saying that it would be good for *you* as well as for your mum and dad if I can help you to *keep your temper*? I can see how it will help them but tell me how it will help *you*. What will be better for *you* when you are able to *keep your temper*?

When/where/with whom/in what situations will it be better? What will be happening/not happening? So, *you won't be getting told off so much*. That sounds good. How does it feel when you get told off? Right, so you're telling me that you won't be feeling angry/fed up/thinking it's unfair when you are able to *take control of your temper*? How will it be instead? Do you think you might *feel a bit proud of yourself because you've taken charge of your temper/you're not calling out so much/you've stopped pushing/shoving*?

Are there already times when you *do manage to keep your temper under control*? Great, so there *are* times when you do it already. Do you have to think about it or do you just *do it automatically*? So sometimes you just know how to do it without even having to think about it. That's going to be very useful; part of you already knows how to control your temper without even thinking about it. Now, let's get some more ideas that you can *try out to see how they work at the time* when you need them. Have you got some ideas about ways to help you *keep your temper*? What could you do/say to yourself/say to them instead?

(At this point, I have found that children will either be quite inventive, suggesting, for example, that they could sing a couple of lines of their favourite tune in their head before answering, or they may come up with something more traditional, such as counting to 10. Sometimes, however, you have to come to the rescue and make a few suggestions, such as: 'One boy I saw the other day suggested he would literally take a step back and take a deep breath before he reacted. He said that would give him time to calm down.' The important thing is to use whatever has most appeal to the child.)

What do you think your mum/dad/grandma will say on hearing that the teacher says *your behaviour has improved so much*?

How surprised will your teacher be when you *are no longer answering back*? Who will be the first person to *notice that there is something different about how you are behaving*? What will be the first thing he or she will notice? What difference will it make to that person?

Scaling

Scaling is a very useful tool in acting as a measure of current behaviour, a means of deciding targets and as a measure of progress (see Chapter 1). Dan, a child who came to see me some years ago, took so well to the idea of scaling his current and desired behaviour that he not only got his family involved but also his enthusiastic form teacher who, each day, would estimate the level he had achieved. Scaling proved to be a remarkable motivator for this child and after only a week his parents and teacher agreed with his estimation that his behaviour had changed from level 1 to level 6 out of 10. He managed a massive turnaround in his behaviour in a matter of only a few weeks along with an interesting change in family dynamics. Previously he had been regularly compared negatively with his angelic younger sister; as Dan's behaviour improved, the sister's declined since she wasn't getting the same amount of attention! The parents then changed their parenting style to giving positive attention (rewarding) for good behaviour in both children, which resulted in increased individual self-esteem and improved family harmony.

Suitable Suggestions

Generally speaking it is probably true, if a little simplistic, to say that you need to consider any negative behaviours and give suggestions for opposite ones. In order for these suggestions to be readily accepted, you ideally need to tap into internal resources that the child will recognise in him or herself. Making use of what the child has told you in conversation, you can suggest in trance that he or she ask the part that knows how to treat their rabbit kindly/gently to help him or her treat classmates more kindly/

gently; the child could ask the part that knows how to concentrate on a PlayStation to concentrate at school and stop disturbing the other children; or the child could ask the part that is amazingly creative at finding excuses for not going to bed to help find ways to surprise the teacher at school by being well-behaved. This slightly paradoxical type of suggestion seems to work quite well in most cases. Suggestions for managing change of any sort are useful, as is the ability to manage disappointment when things don't happen as wanted or expected.

One of the things I have found most helpful when aiming to change behaviour is to ask parents shortly before we start the trance stage of the session to describe some of the qualities they most appreci-ate/enjoy/value about their child. This is a wonderful 'pattern break' for the child who, very probably, has been hearing nothing but negativity for weeks. Imagine how it feels when you hear your mum telling the hypnotherapist, 'When Jake is in a good mood, he can be the most kind and loving boy in the world.' Including reference to this somewhere in the trance state may turn out to be one of the most powerful suggestions you make and one of the best endings can include something along the lines of, 'And just before you open your eyes and come back to the room, I want to remind you that your mum and dad really love you … they think you are the best boy in the world.'

Suitable Inductions

It can often be better to use a confusional induction or at least one that offers choices, preferably double-bind choices, since children with behaviour problems may be inclined to do the opposite of what you ask them to do. Children who tend towards ODD often display polarity responses. It may later transpire that, after one or two sessions, they find they really like the relaxed state and will happily respond to a more relaxing type of induction, especially if they are asked if they want to learn how to do something that not many other children can do.

Before I started treating children with ADHD, I used to think that they would not respond well to gentle progressive relaxation. I believed they would find it boring and react impatiently, but I have found the opposite to be true in nearly every case (although perhaps not always in the first session). It seems that once their bodies start to relax, something inside recognises that this is exactly what they need and they begin to relax quite deeply. Many parents are amazed by how still and calm their child looked during the session.

Working with ADHD or ODD children will certainly keep you on your toes but I have found that on a one-to-one basis these children can be remarkably engaging, creative and keen to change – once you tap into their motivation. You may have to set parameters for the session, but getting them to help you set the rules will normally help them to stick to them. For example, Ben a very bright, quick-minded 13 year old with diagnosed ADHD came to see me with a view to helping him become more relaxed and calm, reduce his tic, control his swearing and generally improve his behaviour and concentration at school. Although I found Ben delightful when we sat face to face, his behaviour was challenging and had been getting him into trouble at school. He took Ritalin when he went to school, but he didn't take it at weekends, holidays or when he came to see me. This meant that he was fidgety and full of nervous energy during our visits, so the two of us set some ground rules: we negotiated the number of times he was allowed to operate the recliner function of the chair; we agreed that he could walk up and down the room 10 times after answering a certain number of questions; we agreed that we – Ben, his foster caregiver (Carolyn), and I – would all take turns speaking without interruption. Setting these rules jointly made it easier for them to be accepted. Ben quickly spotted if I happened to stray from 'the rules', but this was fine as he was quite good-natured when I sometimes pointed out that he was breaking the rules by interrupting. I believe that keeping to specific procedures can be very useful when treating people with ADHD since many sufferers also have obsessions and compulsions involving order, rules and rituals. Keeping the framework of the session fairly constant can be important. I remember Ben asking me in the second session, just as we were about to start the relaxation, if I was going to say 'So Ben …' which I had apparently done in the first session. This phrase had become familiar, as he had listened to my hypnosis recording repeatedly between meetings. After that, the use of 'So Ben' became a little ritual that we used each of the three times he came to see me over a period of a couple of months. The metaphor of the brain as a computer was also used each time so that the program could be adjusted and specific behaviours deleted as his behaviour improved, and, of course, ego strengthening was an integral part of the treatment.

At the time of writing seven or eight months after I first met Ben, the following quote from Carolyn, his foster caregiver, speaks for itself in showing how hypnotherapy treatment can make a real difference. Obviously, the treatment is just one factor; a supportive home and school life are vital ingredients.

Postscript: Ben is continuing to do well at school and at home. I believe that the hypnotism made a big improvement for Ben. His behaviour at school noticeably improved and he has maintained his good behaviour. He changed school in September to the Upper School (a standard move for all pupils) and we were concerned that he may not cope with a larger school that expects more independent learning. However, he coped with the move very well and has been learning at the school very well. At Christmas he received 3 achievement awards at school, something that had been unthinkable before.

Ben no longer listens to the CDs since he does not need to anymore. He listened to them for about 4 or 5 months.

Behaviour Script: Good boy, well done

Age range: approximately 5–9 years

This is a script containing direct and indirect suggestions embedding words of praise. This approach works particularly well when the parent and teacher collaborate in the process.

Good boy (Child's Name) ... you are relaxing so well ... Good boy ... They're nice words aren't they? And the more you hear the words 'Good boy (Child's Name), well done' the more you want to hear those words ... 'Well done' ... You begin to think of ways to hear those words again and hear 'Good boy (Child's Name)' as you *stay in your seat for 10 minutes* ... 'Well done (Child's Name)' when you *listen to your teacher* ... 'Good boy (Child's Name)' when you *want to do what she tells you to do* ... The more you hear the words 'Good boy, well done (Child's Name)' the better you feel in yourself ... When you hear those words, it's like a wonderful colour spreading all over you, all the way through ... Feel it now, how warm is it? How strong is it? Feel it all the way through your mind and body ... You *feel really proud of yourself/feel a sense of satisfaction all the way through* ... as you begin to *think now of other ways to hear those words* ... What can you see yourself doing so that you hear your teacher use those words?... See yourself now doing some of those things ... (leave a pause, adding ... that's right, etc.) ... Then use an appropriate set of commands:

- You are able to stay in your seat.

- You are able to listen when the teacher speaks.

- You are able to stop calling out.

- You are able to get on with your work.

- You are able to stop talking when the teacher talks.

Behaviour Script: Calm and polite

Age range: approximately 9/10–14 years

The script uses a combination of confusion and embedded commands in the induction. Confusion leads the mind to grasp at the next sensible thing it hears and also allows the embedded commands to go unnoticed consciously while they are accepted at the unconscious level.

> ☙ Deliver the first part of the induction at a reasonable pace, perhaps with fewer pauses than normal in order to increase the confusion. Remember to use the stress and intonation of your voice to mark out the italicised embedded commands. ☙

I wouldn't want you to do anything that you don't want to do here today so I don't want you to *let your eyes close* unless that is what you *choose to do yourself* and I don't want you to keep your eyes open and fixed on your hand as you listen to the sound of my voice if you *prefer to let them close all on their own* so if you keep your eyes open while you *fix your attention on your hand and listen to the sound of my voice* that will be fine … but if on the other hand… you prefer to *concentrate on your thoughts* and *let your eyes close* as you look at that hand that will be fine too. … I wouldn't want you to *let your eyes close* unless you feel … as you really *begin to feel more relaxed* … that you really want to let those eyes close … and as you find it harder and harder to know whether the eyes *are more relaxed* than the arms or whether the legs *are more relaxed* than the arms … you might want to think about whether you are generally comfortable enough with the way things are and whether *you are comfortable* enough with yourself.

I think *there is* a part of you that is uncomfortable with getting into trouble and doesn't *know how to change all that* … and I also know there is a part of you that wants to *feel more comfortable* than the uncomfortable part … and that this part of you is the one that can *find a way to get through the school day more quietly and comfortably* … finding it easier to *choose to behave the polite way* than the other way … finding it natural to *answer questions in a pleasant way* … and *finding it strangely unnatural and difficult to be rude* … it almost seems that the part of you that *used* to want to be comfortable with being rude has found the right way to be *un*comfortable with being rude … and that the way left is to *be comfortable being polite* … it's funny how the more you try to remember to be rude the more you *remember how to be polite to your teacher* ... and for longer and longer each day you seem to really *want to be friendly and helpful* ... and the more you try to be rude the more difficult it is to remember that old way of talking ... and as *you enjoy being friendly and helpful more and more each day* somehow the part of you that *wants to be comfortable with that feels more and more settled and calm* ... almost but not quite ready ... or are *you?* ... *Quite ready now to go deeper now* into this *new way* ... or is it already an *old* way of thinking and feeling good about yourself? ... *feeling so good now ... feeling so comfortable now with the idea that you are a special person with lots to offer to others around ... feeling good about you ... feeling good about who you are* ... able to *let your real polite self have a chance to show itself at school as well as at home* ... able to *enjoy doing so well and like hearing the praise from your teachers* ... able to *enjoy the surprise on your mum's face when she hears the teacher say how very well you are doing right now* ... and *you are doing this so well ... you are so good at concentrating in a very special way* right now is the time for you to begin to drift back to the room now ... feeling proud that you knew how to do this ... and find that you have been able to *make some changes on the inside* ... that will show the world on the outside just *how good you are all the way through* ... so coming back now I'm wondering ... and maybe *you're* wondering too ... what will be the *first way* that you will *notice the change in you that helps you to feel better about you* and what will be the first way that your mum will notice and will it, I wonder ... be your mum or your dad or your friend who first sees that little difference in you ... or will it be so big that *nobody* could miss it? ... I'm looking forward to seeing you next time to know how it was ... and who it was who first noticed that difference ... and how that made you feel ... so as I slowly count from 1 to 10 and your eyelids feel lighter and lighter and *you feel better and better* ... I wonder whether with each number you *see a picture of yourself acting a little differently in class.*

1 ... see yourself feeling better about how you behave ... 2 ... hear your teacher saying 'Well Done' ... 3 ... you forget about those old uncomfortable ways ... 4 ... you feel more and more confident about behaving well ... 5 ... you are more and more able to think before you speak ... 6 ... you enjoy being you ... 7 ... you have more self-respect ... 8 ... you enjoy respecting yourself and others around you ... 9 ... you respect you and you respect them and they respect you and now I expect 10 ... you are right back here with me ... well done.

Behaviour Script: Calm and well behaved in class

Age range: approximately 8/9–12 years

The script uses a combination of confusion and embedded commands to combat hyperactivity. Confusion leads the mind to grasp at the next sensible thing it hears and also allows the embedded commands to be unnoticed consciously while they are accepted at the unconscious level. Adapt the script to include relevant suggestions as appropriate.

(Child's Name) I'd like you to cup your hands upward lightly on your lap and then choose to look into the centre of them … *really* look at, I mean … as you look at them in this different way … very, very still and very, very focused … I'd like you to notice how when you look straight in the centre you can see both of them at the same time … you can notice which fingers are staying very, very still … not moving at all … at the same time as noticing fingers that have tiny little movements all by themselves.

I know there is a part of you that doesn't want to *stop moving around and feeling uncomfortable* and I know too there's a special part of you *(Child's Name)* that wants to … *relax* and *feel very comfortable* as you look at your hands … and there may be a part that doesn't *yet* know how to … *listen to other people* … and there's another special part of you that wants to *listen carefully* to what I say … and the part of you that wants to *relax now* … may be the part of you that makes your eyelids feel very heavy … or it may be the other part of you that doesn't *yet* know how to *relax more quickly* that makes them *feel so heavy* … maybe they *feel so heavy* that they *want to close sooner* … or later … and I think maybe that part ☞ **If the eyes are still open, include the next phrase in brackets.** ☞ (that wants to concentrate so hard that they stay open) is the part of you that wants you to … *take control of your behaviour at school* …

And while you are thinking of the many different ways … you can control your behaviour … this special part of your inner mind can *decide (Child's Name) right now to* … do it in *the right way* for you because you are a very special boy who … does *know the right way to behave at school and at home.*

I wonder which way your special inner mind will *decide now first* … will it be to *do what the teacher tells you the first time and get on with your work*? … Or, will it be this second to decide to *stay calm and refuse to retaliate/react/fight back* if people tease? … Or will it be the first, second or third second that it decides to *stop the calling out?* … And I wonder if your teacher, your dad, your mum or you will be most pleased and surprised that you *stay (Child's Name) out of trouble* … and do the right thing, in the right way, and what is left is for you to do it right away, at the right time and if you do everything at the right time … I wonder what will be left for you to do to surprise yourself and *surprise your mum* with how this part of you with all its special abilities to … *be thoughtful and kind* … can find so many ways for you to … *enjoy yourself* being very good and very special?

And I wonder … when you come back to see me next time … how you will tell me … that you knew automatically that it was right for you to calm down … *quiet down in class* and find that you really enjoyed your teacher noticing that you were making an effort to *stop disturbing other people.*

But just before we finish today I'd like you to concentrate very hard on your hands ☞ **If the child's eyes are closed, say instead, 'I want you to imagine you can still see those hands on your lap and concentrate very hard.'** ☞ until you can see a picture appear of you … just like in a film/movie … of you

201

with all those changes made ... you are sitting so comfortably still for ages and ages ... you look so calm and relaxed ... can you see how confident you look as you are listening so hard to what the teacher is saying? ... Hey ... is that you putting your hand up to answer the question? ... It is (Child's Name) ... It's *you* answering the question ... and now look ... when the teacher says it's time to do some writing ... is it you who is the first one to get down to it? ... Well done ... fantastic ... somehow the more you were even to try to put off starting, the more *you feel you just have to do it straightaway* ... and one more picture now ... this is almost the best I think ... there are some children trying to disturb you ... digging you in the arm ... trying to take your rubber/pen and you are just not taking any notice of them at all ... aren't you just fantastic! ... You are totally ignoring them and just getting on with your work ... amazing!

So, now I think it's time for you to come back to the room ... coming more and more awake ... not that you were asleep ... coming fully wide awake at the count of 10 ... fully aware that you know how to concentrate your attention completely ... eyes wide open ... fully aware that you ... have a stretch ... can be confidently calm and calmly confident that you can concentrate in this brilliant new way ... well done.

Behaviour script: Congratulations on progress

Age range: approximately 5/6–8 years

The script uses a combination of congratulations on progress achieved and embedded commands to continue the good work.

I'd like to congratulate you because you have already been able to *cut down the calling out (Child's Name) ... and I know that* mum and dad are very pleased that you have already *cut down the calling out* and are able to *stop getting out of your seat.*

Now inside your mind did you know that there is a special control room with special switches and controls for all the things you do? ... for example, there is a control for letting you know when you are hungry and thirsty and there are controls for calling out and getting out of your seat ... Imagine that you can see this control room on the television screen of your mind ... Have a look around and notice the different dials and switches. Can you see? Look, there's hunger/thirst/being helpful/behaving well ... Now have a look at the one for 'calling out' ... See what number it is set on ... Number 10 is what you used to do (calling out a lot) and number 0 is not calling out at all ... See what number you're at now ... and decide what number you can turn down the dial to so *you automatically stop calling out altogether/getting out of your seat* ... Great ... Well done, *(Child's Name)*.

Now change the channel and see *(Child's Name)* at school, sitting in his seat ... *getting on with your work quietly, (Child's Name)* ... *See yourself enjoying your work now …* Look at your teacher's face … she looks so surprised and pleased that *you are in control, (Child's Name) …* now you have been able to *stop calling out* and *stop getting out of your seat …* Look at the other children too! They really like it now you are not getting into trouble … It *feels good,* doesn't it? … You *feel good about yourself now you are calm and confident.*

Behaviour Script: Manage change and disappointment

Age range: approximately 9/10 years upward

Have you ever looked into a kaleidoscope? One of those tubes that you hold up to your eye … where you see wonderful patterns of different shapes and sizes … amazing colours, and when you turn the tube with your fingers you change the pattern … the shapes rearrange themselves … go on do it now in your mind … What can you see? Look at the shapes and colours and the fantastic pattern …now turn it a bit and change the pattern … *notice the changes … how easily you made them.*

Now I'd like you to look into the kaleidoscope of your life … look in it and see some of the situations in your life … some you like … and some you like a little less … perhaps some are a bit disappointing … look at the way you handle things … some situations are easy to handle and some need a bit more thought, don't they? … Sometimes things happen and we can't change them … they're not our choice and we have to live with them but … here's the thing … maybe we can't change the situation but we can *change the way we think about them … change how we feel about them* and *change what we say about them* … and when we do that, *all kinds of things can feel a little easier … you cope a bit more easily … you can feel a bit stronger.*

So, since this is your own kaleidoscope why not experiment a bit … look into it and see that situation that used to upset you … and try changing your thoughts about it and … as you do … turn the tube around/shake the tube and see the difference it makes … try out something new … try out saying something different … try out shrugging your shoulders and smiling and *notice how that changes your feelings* … try out the thought … 'perhaps it will turn out for the best' … or … 'maybe something good will happen'. ☞ **Include a guided visualisation of the child coping positively and confidently with changing circumstances specific to the individual situation.** ☜

And I want you to know that here in this special state of mind … calm and relaxed … you can focus easily … and because you can focus more easily than before … you can *change that focus more easily than before* … and being aware how *a big change can happen easily* … simply by turning something round … simply by changing the view … you can begin to *look at change in a rather different way … change your point of view* … so from now on you will find that *you are able to cope with ever-changing situations more and more comfortably … cope more and more easily* … you will find that *you are able to pick yourself up when things don't go the way you wanted* … far more easily than you did in the past … you pick yourself up and *get going again … you are more positive and hopeful that things can go well* … things will go well … you have new opportunities to try out different things … different ways at looking at things … congratulations … well done … time to re-orientate to the room … feeling wonderful and wider and wider awake as I count to 10.

Chapter Thirteen

Learning and Exams

Who is Likely to Present for Hypnotherapy Treatment?

Children who:

- do well at coursework but are anxious when faced with tests and exams.

- underachieve or do not meet their parents' expectations.

- need help with focus, concentration and organisation of thinking and learning either in class or with doing homework.

- display several of the symptoms of Attention Deficit Hyperactivity Disorder (ADHD), whether or not they fulfil all the criteria for a diagnosis.

- display several of the symptoms of Dyslexia, whether or not they fulfil all the criteria for a diagnosis.

- lack confidence in their ability and have low self-esteem.

- have teachers who are unsympathetic to them for one reason or another and this affects their schoolwork negatively.

- have anxiety problems.

- have emotional problems.

- are suffering from school phobia and so may be behind with their work, at least in part, because of infrequent attendance.

The majority of children I have seen for the above problems have been quite keen to be helped and happy to cooperate. However, a few have had the feeling of being unfairly criticised by teachers, parents or both and so have started out by being slightly uncooperative. The first requirement is to 'get them on side' or you will get nowhere at all. See Chapters 1 and 12 for discussions of this topic and for solution-focused questions to help win them over. When problems arise from lack of concentration, it may be preferable to adapt normal practice to offer a number of short sessions rather than one or two of customary length. I also find that supporting CDs provide invaluable help in these cases, either your own or from a publisher (see the Useful Resources section).

In taking a case history, it is important to discover whether the child is suffering from emotional problems and/or anxiety as these may be at the centre of his or her difficulties with academic work. Check for causes such as bullying, family or marital disharmony, grief, depression or physical ill health, as these will all need to be addressed before, or sometimes concurrently with, the more academic issues. You will find discussions of some of these problems in other chapters in this book. The current chapter concentrates on dealing with matters more directly linked to the learning process. Other issues, such as depression or grief, school phobia or problems arising from dysfunctional family relationships, may well be underlying factors in lack of concentration, focus and self-belief but their treatment requires far more in-depth discussion than is appropriate here. However, it should be kept in mind that in certain cases, depending on the experience and training of the practitioner, the right course of action will be to refer to other professionals who specialise in the areas of specific concern. When using hypnotherapy to help children cope better with the learning process, their learning environment, or with tests and exams, it is axiomatic that ego-strengthening approaches should be a vital component of your treatment strategy.

Accelerated Learning

Awareness of some basic principles of learning will aid your choice of hypnotic suggestions to help the child at a very practical level. Many accelerated learning techniques are simple to learn and very helpful to teach pupils and students of any abilities. They are particularly useful when children may be struggling with a more verbal approach. It is possible that if these children were to experiment with visual and kinaesthetic strategies, it could bring about a marked positive change in their performance. The following list provides basic concepts, some that will be familiar and others not, that are useful to incorporate into scripts when appropriate for your particular young client. I have selected a few concepts that in my former existence as a teacher I found especially helpful.

Helpful Concepts in Accelerated Learning

Use all the senses

The brain learns in words, pictures, feelings and actions. It likes to read things, to hear things, to say and do things too. Sometimes, it even learns using associations with tastes and smells!

It helps us to remember information if we bring as many of the senses as possible into the learning process. Some children tend towards a style of learning that is more visual, auditory or kinaesthetic so if they are having difficulties with processing and remembering information in one medium, it can be effective to encourage them to make use of a different, preferred medium as well. For example, reading the words aloud or making a diagram or a picture on the page, or even in the imagination if a child is not allowed to write in the book, may serve as a memory prompt for children who are experiencing reading issues. Pictures that are colourful, funny, memorable, uniquely meaningful (or even rude!) can be particularly helpful.

One way to strengthen learning and memory is to use colour when reading and when writing notes. Use brightly coloured pens to highlight words, pictures or ideas with **connections** in the **same** colour so that you form associations between things. Use coloured pens and squiggly lines to connect up linked ideas and concepts.

Tactile/kinaesthetic strategies include having children write things down, trace words or drawings with their fingers while they memorise, or write key words and phrases on index cards and order them into groups, or type up notes on a computer, to name just a few.

Associations

The brain likes to use associations and remember things in groups rather than in isolation so it is useful to find ways to link information together, for example, through Mind Maps, linked stories and pictures, metaphors and funny mnemonics.

Mind Maps™

The use of colourful Mind Maps is an excellent way to make notes of things we need to remember since they emphasise connections between concepts that reflect the way the brain stores information in neural networks. Buzan (2005) has a book for children in addition to the many he has written for adults.

Mnemonics

The following is an example of a mnemonic that helps you to remember how to spell the word **DIARROHEA** (British spelling): **D**ash **I**n **A** **R**eal **R**ush **O**r **H**ave **E**mbarrassing **A**ccident.

Linked story

An example of a linked story is to use the child's bedroom as a way to remember apparently unrelated items such as the names and order of the wives of Henry VIII. 'Imagine you are standing outside your bedroom door when you notice that the name of Catherine of Aragon is written in enormous letters all over the door nearly as big as you. Can you see it? What colour is it? Can you see a picture of her too? Good, now open the door and what do you see immediately in front of you? Okay, your dressing table. Put a picture of Anne Boleyn on your dressing table.' (If you want to be gruesome, you could have her holding her beheaded head in her hands with her name on it!) Continue around the room in one direction, adding pictures or names as you go with frequent backtracking to start from the beginning again to reinforce the memory.

Baroque music

Having music composed between 1700–1750, such as Bach, Vivaldi or Mozart, playing quietly in the background can help increase calm, concentration and creativity. It is theorised that this may be partly because the rhythm of this style of music tends to encourage the alpha brainwave rhythm and partly because it stimulates the creative and logical processes of the brain to work in harmony. If you can't persuade a child to try this style of music, any gentle relaxing music **without words** to distract would probably work quite well (see the Useful Resources section for relaxing music specifically to induce a sense of calm and well-being).

Working in short bursts

Working in short concentrated bursts will usually be more effective than expecting a child to sit and study for protracted periods of time. Twenty to 30 minutes study with a 5-minute 'move-around break' followed by another 20 minutes study is ideal.

The Primary/Recency Effect

This theory suggests that we have better recall of information when it is the first and the last that we receive – the beginning and end of a chapter, talk or lesson. By giving ourselves breaks, we increase the occurrence of beginnings and endings with their first and last bits of information.

Review

Recall is increased dramatically if we review information on a frequent and regular basis; therefore, just before we take a break, we should close our eyes and recall what we have been learning, and each time we return to study after a 5- or 10-minute break, we should test ourselves on what we learned before the break.

Active reading

Reading actively increases participation in the process and more participation will increase understanding, retention and recall. See the script 'Improve your reading for information skills' and related handout for children for more detail about active reading.

When you are working with children concerning their homework, it is important to discuss aims and objectives thoroughly with parents to make sure that they are in agreement with any approaches you suggest, particularly when introducing ideas such as working in short bursts and taking breaks or having music playing as a background to study.

Attention Deficit Hyperactivity Disorder

Children showing attention deficit signs may tend to be:

*   dreamy/disorganised/forgetful/inattentive.

They may tend to:

*   have difficulty in listening/lack concentration/fail to follow instructions, probably because they were not listening or concentrating in the first place/lose things/take a long time to start tasks/fail to finish tasks/avoid homework.

The hyperactivity aspect of ADHD is discussed and suitable scripts are suggested in Chapter 12. This present chapter provides scripts that focus on helping with the attention deficit aspect of the disorder. One of the most effective ways to help children with the above problems is to elicit occasions when they *do* find that they are able to concentrate for long periods of time – for example, when they are playing on their computer or listening to music. When they are in the trance state we can 'anchor' that behaviour and 'map it across' to other desired situations, such as the classroom or doing homework. The scripts 'Listening and getting started' and 'Concentrate and stay focused' use this technique. Scripts that help these children to develop the belief that they are able to change their behaviour and build their self-esteem will also have a significant potential impact.

Dyslexia

Dyslexia is Greek word meaning 'difficulty with words', and it is a condition that primarily affects reading and spelling. (Dyscalculia refers to problems with numerical skills and Dyspraxia generally refers to problems with fine and gross motor skills.) Dyslexia sufferers may also experience difficulties in processing visual and/or auditory information and they will normally also have short-term memory problems. Difficulties may be apparent in spoken as well as written language. In speech, finding the right word can be tricky; there may be a lot of 'thingamies', 'you knows' and 'stuff' plus unfinished utterances, which may make the speaker sound a bit incoherent.

Research suggests that these specific language-processing difficulties occur in the left hemisphere of the brain and there is considerable evidence for a genetic disposition since Dyslexia tends to run in families. However, no single gene has yet been found to be responsible for the condition. Neither is there a single worldwide accepted definition of exactly what Dyslexia is, so it is often used as an umbrella term (as is Dyspraxia) to cover a wide variety of specific learning difficulties. Estimates used to suggest that more boys than girls were affected but more recent thinking finds that these estimates may possibly have derived from teacher 'referral bias' rather than there being any true gender difference. Boys may be referred more often for assessment because of a tendency to cope with difficulty and 'perceived failure in a display of indifference and disruptive behaviour' whereas girls may 'do their utmost to avoid unwanted notice' (Everatt and Zabell, 2000).

Dyslexia is not linked to culture, social background or intelligence and it is encountered across all levels of academic ability. Interestingly, it has been found that many people with Dyslexia have strong creative abilities and are innovative, lateral thinkers who tend to think outside the box. This probably accounts for the fact that many hugely successful entrepreneurs and artists number among the Dyslexic population. These people often did not enjoy school and certainly didn't shine there, probably because their creative and intuitive intelligence was not appreciated in a system that values highly traditional, academic, analytical and written skills.

Possible Primary Symptoms

- Difficulty in reading and writing.
- Inaccuracy in spelling.
- Writing letters and digits back to front.
- Inaccurate comprehension (probably caused by misreading).
- Difficulty with the phonic approach to spelling, e.g., mapping sounds onto clusters of letters.

Possible Secondary Symptoms

- Generally poor organisational skills.
- Little awareness or management of time.
- Poor short-term memory and concentration.
- Difficulty in planning, organising and analytical thinking.
- Difficulty with processing or producing sequential information.
- Low self-image.

Having Dyslexia does not necessarily mean that children cannot perform the above processes well; rather that they will have ongoing difficulties with varying levels of severity in carrying out all or some of the aspects. The specific child's individual strengths and weaknesses will play a part in this, as will the amount of relevant teaching, support and encouragement received both at school and at home. While there are a wide variety of symptoms experienced by those with Dyslexia, there is one that many Dyslexics share: poor self-image. They *feel* stupid because they don't process information as easily or as quickly as others and their poor school results usually reinforce this feeling and low opinion of themselves. They may suffer teasing from other pupils and even be insensitively handled by certain teachers not well trained to recognise Dyslexia or deal appropriately with children with specific learning difficulties.

What are Appropriate Aims for Hypnotherapy?

- Boost self-image and self-confidence.

- Discover and emphasise individual strengths, e.g., the ability to concentrate for long periods of time on PlayStations!

- Get clients to understand that the difficulties experienced do not come from stupidity.

- Discard/ignore unhelpful negative beliefs and opinions of self or others.

- Help them to *manage* their difficulties. Do not suggest that you can 'cure' them.

- Improve listening and concentration skills.

- Strengthen perseverance.

- Improve courage/confidence to ask for help and extra time when needed.

- Teach the NLP visual strategy for easier spelling, which helps people whose preference for learning may be visual rather than auditory.

Important Aspects of Delivery

- Use all the senses (visual, auditory, kinaesthetic) in your suggestions.

- Speak slowly, use lots of repetition, use lots of pauses. Keep the sessions brief.

- Appeal to the client's colourful and creative mind.

Learning Script: Listening and getting started

Age range: approximately 8/10–14 years according to how you choose to adapt specific vocabulary and ideas

In the third paragraph of the script, there is a reference to the fact that the child listens to music during spare time and this is used as an anchor for auditory focus. Therefore, it is essential that you establish in your pre-trance discussion that the child does, indeed, enjoy listening to music. If not, find an appropriate activity and adapt the script accordingly. You can also incorporate relevant suggestions from the 'Concentrate and stay focused' script.

> Settle yourself down comfortably while you *listen and let your eyes close* … easily and naturally balancing the weight in both sides of your body … and drift off to some lovely, relaxing place where you can … *feel very, very comfortable, comfortable in yourself, comfortable about yourself in every way* … as you listen to the sound of my voice the amazing thing is … that the more intently/ closely you listen to the sound of my voice … the more comfortable and calm and relaxed you feel … The more calm and relaxed your body becomes … the more calm and focused your mind becomes … and you just enjoy feeling calm and focused on the inside … calm and focused on the outside … calm and focused inside out … all the way through.

(Child's Name), you told me that you want me to help you *listen and get down to things more easily* at school and *get down to your homework in a very focused way* ... and isn't it nice to know that here ... with me ... the best way to listen is in a kind of listening dream where you can be very creative indeed while you *focus your mind* ... and we know ... do we not, that *you are very creative.*

Remember you told me that when you're listening to music on your headphones that *your mind is fully focused on the music* ... Why not drift back to one of those times ... Just be there now in your mind ... put on your headphones ... yes, that's it ... whenever you put on your headphones ... you are completely tuned in/focused ... Brilliant ... Notice how it feels when you are listening so intently ... Now let yourself double that intense listening experience as you take a deep breath ... yes, that's it ... and strengthen that feeling right now and let it spread all over you ... Wonderful ... I wonder how it would be if you were to just *double that again right now* ... Great ... *focused on the sound* ... just as you were then ... just as you are now ... just as you *will* be whenever you want to *focus and concentrate on what your teacher is saying* ... and I want you to know that from now on when you are in class and the teacher is talking ... you will feel this urge to put on your imaginary headphones and *listen intently to what the teacher is saying* ... and as you listen ... you will *feel so good about you* ... *feel so positive about you* ... The more you *listen to what the teacher is saying* ... *the more positive you feel about you.*

And just listening and relaxing right now this minute ... *you are drawn like an amazing magnet to the ideas I give you* to help you listen ... to help you focus ... and to help you learn more easily now ... So ready now ... from now on ... whenever you are in the classroom ... you have an urge to put on your imaginary headphones and *listen closely to every word the teacher says* ... and because you listen so well ... you understand better than you ever have before.

In class when you are listening to instructions for what to do next ... you focus and *repeat them silently in your head* and you will *naturally find them easier to remember* ... say that to yourself now ... *I will listen to instructions and repeat them in my head* ... ... That's it.

You get down to things straightaway ... say that to yourself now ... I will get down to things straightaway ... ... That's right.

Then do a little bit at a time ... you *get down to the first little bit straightaway* ... when you do a little bit at a time it makes it so much easier for you to *achieve what you want to achieve* ... say that to yourself now ... I will *do a little bit at a time* ... ... Brilliant.

You *stay focused and you keep track of time* ... say that to yourself now ... I will *stay focused* and I will *keep track of time* ... ... That's it.

214

Sometimes you will want to *check the time* and set yourself a time limit to *do what you have been asked to do* … say that to yourself now … I will check the time and I will set myself a time limit to do exactly what I've been asked to do … … … Yes.

Now you can get even more creative … just transport yourself into the classroom … be there now … sitting in your seat … and put on your imaginary headphones that help you to listen … *really* listen I mean … you *listen so attentively to your teacher that you absorb every word they say* … just following every word … you are *drawn like a magnet to listen* … just as you are listening to the sound of my voice right now … you repeat all instructions to yourself in your head so you *know just what you have to do and you do it straight off* … and you *feel so positive* do you not? … Notice how … when other children are trying to distract/disturb you and get you to talk to them … the more you want to *listen to the teacher* … The harder they try to distract/disturb you … the more you *focus on your work.*

Now … go through this again very, very quickly in your mind with *each teacher* … *with each lesson* … and nod your head when you come to the end of the day … ☺ **Give the child plenty of time to do this.** ☺ and notice how you *feel so very good* about you … *how proud you feel* of yourself … Now do it for the next day … Brilliant …. Now, do it for the next day (until you have gone through the whole school week).

Well done … and now you've focused so hard and done so fantastically well … it's time for you to come back to full alert awareness of the room as I count from 1 to 10 … each number bringing you wider and wider awake and back here feeling positive, confident and delighted with how very well you've done today.

Learning Script: Concentrate and stay focused

Age range: approximately 10 years upward according to how you choose to adapt specific vocabulary and ideas

☺ **Elicit in your pre-trance talk an activity in which the child is focused and confident so that you can make use of it in the third paragraph of the script.** ☺

Settle yourself in the chair and find the most comfortable position for you to listen … and as you do … I want you to focus on that light switch over there … and as you listen and as you focus totally on that light switch … I'd like you to observe whether it becomes fuzzy and blurred or whether the outline becomes more and more defined … and while you're deciding whether *it's fuzzy and blurred* or *the outline gets more and more defined* … I'm wondering whether your eyelids feel really, really light … or whether they *feel really, really heavy* … or indeed whether they will *become even heavier and heavier* … so heavy in fact that they will *want to close straightaway* or whether that will just happen in a little while ... or not at all ... as *your focus becomes more and more intense* and your amazing mind is more and more focused on accepting all the helpful suggestions you told me you *really want to follow right now* so whether you *let your eyes close ... easily and naturally ... to become even more comfortable ...* or whether you try hard to keep them open for a little bit longer really doesn't matter at all ... whichever you choose will be perfect for you ... so long as you *feel very, very comfortable, comfortable in yourself, comfortable about yourself in every way.*

(Child's Name), you told me you want me to help you *concentrate your thinking and stay focused* at school and help you *do your homework in a very focused and organised way* ... and isn't it nice to know that here ... with me ... you have already demonstrated that *you can focus and concentrate brilliantly* ... and the best way to listen is in a kind of daydream where you can be very creative indeed while you *focus your mind* ... and we know ... do we not ... that *you are very creative.*

Remember you told me that when you're skateboarding/running/dancing *your mind is fully focused on what you're doing* ... so drift back to one of those skateboarding/running/dancing times where you were so focused ... that *everything goes just right* ... Just be there now in your mind ... *you are completely tuned in ... really focused* ... you *see what you need to do* and you just *do it naturally* ... everything is working out right ... yes, that's it ... brilliant ... hear the word *focus* in your head ... Notice those wonderful confident feelings you have at the same time ... are they warm or cool? ... What colour are they? ... Are they moving or still? ... Now take a deep breath ... yes, that's it ... and *strengthen that feeling right now* and *let it spread all over you* ... wonderful ... now do it again and *double those confident focused feelings* ... each time you take a deep breath ... you strengthen those feelings and *you are confident and focused* ... a great way to be ... I want you to know that every time you take a deep breath ... your whole mind and body will remember exactly how to *be at your most confident and focused* ... just as you were then ... just as you are now ... just as you *will* be whenever you want to *focus and concentrate on your work ... and you really will want to focus and concentrate all of your attention on whatever task you are doing at the time.*

And with each breath you take ... see it filling your body ... feel it filling your mind with calm and confidence ... that's right, the colour spreading all around now as confident thoughts come into your mind ... each breath balancing your mind and body ... begin to breathe any unwanted colour of tension or self-doubt right away from your mind.

That's right ... that's brilliant ... now you're ready to go inside your dreaming mind ... and find yourself in your classroom now ... look at the black/white board ... and check the hidden, mistaken, unhelpful beliefs and messages about yourself on the board ... maybe you've never consciously noticed them before because they were hiding behind the words ... but when you look

216

closely you can perhaps see some mistaken negative messages … really, really silly things … some people see messages that tell them that they can't do this or that, or they're not clever enough to understand … you know the kind of thing … that is completely mistaken thinking … if you should find any negative message … even one … I want you right now this minute to *wipe it off/wash it off/scrub it off immediately.* ☜ **Give the child plenty of time to do it.** ☞ That's it … brilliant … well done … but your job is only half done … now it's time to write up your positive, confident, focused messages instead … so you can think positively and confidently about yourself … so please pick up the pen/chalk … make it a brightly coloured one … and write on the board as I give you some positive and very powerful messages that will actually help you to … *focus and concentrate on the task at hand* and … as you write … they will *become a very real part of you* and as you *look closely at the board every day* … your new beliefs get stronger and stronger … and how soon will it be before these new beliefs are no longer your *new beliefs* because *you are so at home with them* they feel as if *they have always been there* … will always *be a part of you.*

So, let's go … *I am bright and I can focus my mind … I can concentrate and learn new things very well … I know I have strengths and I will remember them … I am learning to be more confident in my ability to focus and concentrate every day … It's getting easier to concentrate for longer and longer each day.*

Good … well done … now every time in class when you look at the board, you will *remember these powerful beliefs* … and even when you just go inside your mind at home and see that board … you will feel confident, calm and in control of your thinking … The amazing thing is … that the more you *focus your attention on that board … the more calm and focused your mind becomes* … and the more calm and focused you become … the more you just *enjoy that feeling* … calm and focused on the inside … calm and focused on the outside … calm and focused inside out and all the way through.

So just before we finish I'd like you to see yourself on your mental television screen during the following days and weeks in the classroom … have a look and just notice what is different about you … Is it the way you look so alert? … Is it the way you are sitting? … Is it the way your attention is so concentrated on what you are doing? … Is it that when you look at the board, you are noticing the positive messages about you? … I wonder which of your teachers will be the first to notice the difference in you. … and how soon will it be that they notice the difference in the quality of your work? … And which will please them most, I wonder … will it be that *you are concentrating so much more* or will it be that the quality of your work has improved so much? … And I wonder what will please *you* the most? … And I wonder what will please your mum/dad the most? … And I wonder who, out of all of you, is the most proud of you? … I certainly hope it's you … because you were the one who just somehow knew deep down inside … that *you certainly do have the ability to focus and to concentrate and to enjoy being you.*

217

So, wonderful … in a few moment's time, I'm going to ask you to come right back to the present moment only as quickly as you have stored all of the brilliant feelings of focus and concentration inside … and as you do … you will notice how positive and confident you feel right now and as I count from 1 to 10, each ascending number will help you come back to the room feeling wide, wide awake … Any heavy sleepy feelings will be lifted from you … you will be wide, wide awake with a wonderful calm and focused feeling all over.

Learning Script: Improve your studying/reading for information skills (Homework)

Age range: approximately 12 years upward

And feeling comfortably relaxed now … it's easy to drift off in your mind to the internet … go to your favourite search engine and type in the words 'Study Tips' … and look at the site that comes up … the main heading says Study Tips and down the side there are some separate headings … click on the one that says 'Study Times' and look at what it says … right … here we go.

Work for 20 to 30 minutes maximum at a time and then give yourself a 5-minute break to have a stretch, move around, get a glass of water, eat a piece of fruit if you want … this will help you *focus even more when you come back to study* … time the break for 5 minutes exactly and you will *find yourself really keen to get back to your work* … each time you come back to your work … you have a strong urge to *test yourself on what you learnt before the break* and each time you test yourself … you will remember more and more … *remember more and more easily* too … and how soon will it be, I wonder before your body and your mind seem to *remember exactly when that 5 minutes has passed* before you even look at the clock … and your feet are taking you back to where you were studying … and your hands are picking up that book and you are already testing yourself on what you know now that you didn't know before … well done.

So, now look at those other headings and click on 'Ways to organise your reading and learning' … here we go.

Before you even start to read a chapter … see if you can guess what the main ideas are going to be from the title of the chapter … and as you read … you can notice if your guess was right … the more you do it the better your guesses become … and the better your guesses become … the more you *enjoy doing it* … and getting that satisfying feeling inside.

Read the first paragraph *first* and then read the *last* paragraph *next* … because these are the paragraphs that often give you the most important information … then look at any diagrams and pictures because they help to make things clear.

When you begin the chapter, you always remember to ask yourself what you want to learn from reading this particular chapter … make notes of the questions you want to find answers to … and as you read, you will *notice the answers as you read* and … as you *notice the answers straightaway* … it may even seem to you that the answers are highlighted in colour on the page, and they stand out so clearly you couldn't miss them if you tried … you will *remember those answers so easily and effortlessly* … it may even surprise you how easily they seem to be fixed in your mind … you seem to *see those answers in bright colour in your mind's eye.*

Then go back to the beginning again and as you read and find useful information … if it is your own book … use a bright highlighter pen to focus and highlight the important information … not only in your mind's eye, but use the highlighter on the page too … (If it isn't your own book, you can use the highlighter in your mind's eye.)

Then go through again and make notes of the key/important words and phrases … I don't know whether you will want to draw a picture or a diagram instead of words … either will be absolutely fine … and when you do them in colour too you will find you *remember them* even better … whichever colour you choose will be perfect for you … whichever picture you draw will be perfect for you.

It's time to log off now … but I want you to know … that each time that you read in this way, you will *become more and more confident that this is a good way for you to learn* … in fact you will not only *become more confident in organising your reading and learning* … you will *become more confident in other ways too … more and more confident in your ability … more and more confident in yourself* … more and more confident in your ability to *read and learn in a relaxed and confident way* … and as *you are becoming more relaxed and confident in so many different ways* … you notice yourself noticing that you seem to *be happier* in so many different ways too.

Right now it's time for you to come back to the room … feeling absolutely great … feeling full of positivity … and really *keen to try out new ideas that will improve your ability to study easily and effectively* … becoming aware as I count from 1 to 10 that all the energy is coming back into your body as your mind becomes super alert and your eyes will open only as quickly as you know you have learned something really important for you that will enable you to *become a brilliant learner* … and as the days and the weeks go by I wonder just what will be the signs that *you are really enjoying this active way of taking charge of your learning* and who will be the people who first *notice the change in the quality of your work*? Well done … fantastic.

Handout for children to support the 'Improve your studying/Reading for information skills' script

Improve your reading for information

Work 20 / 30 mins

5-min break

Stretch / walk around / drink water / eat a piece of fruit

Go back to your work

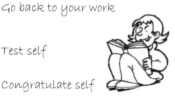

Test self

Congratulate self

Read chapter title   Guess what's going to be in the chapter

 Read first para and last para

Look at any diagrams

Look for important info and highlight it in colour

Close your eyes and see it in colour in your head

Make notes of important info / use pics and diagrams

You are learning more

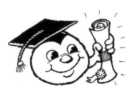 You are becoming more confident every day in every way!

Congratulations!

220

Spelling strategy conversational script

Age range: adaptable to any age

This is based on the NLP Spelling Strategy devised by Robert Dilts* who, observing what good spellers do naturally, came up with a visual strategy to help people who had difficulties with spelling. This strategy has been found useful with children who seem to be using mainly auditory and kinaesthetic approaches rather than visual ones. It uses a visual rather than a phonic approach. It involves getting children to use their eye movements in a way that ensures they can visualise more easily. The prompt script suggests looking up to their left but with left-handed children you may find that telling them to look up to their right works better for them. Practise using this with two or three people before you use it with a client to check you are completely familiar with the procedure.

Procedure

Before you start, ask the child for a word that he or she always has great difficulty in spelling and, using a board pen, write it clearly in big, bold, colourful lower case letters on a piece of paper. (Make certain that you have the right spelling! If you are not sure, you and the child can look the word up in the dictionary together.)

Prompt script

Close your eyes and think of something that makes you feel really good, maybe when you are pleased with yourself because you have done something really well. Got that nice feeling inside? Good.

Now still with this good feeling inside, open your eyes and look at the word you want to learn to spell. (Show the client the word you have written down.)

Now close your eyes (or look at the wall over there) and look upward and over to your left and imagine seeing this word written in large letters on a white board. See it in your favourite colour and make it nice and bright and clear. Can you see it? Is it very clear? How big is it? What colour is it? Excellent.

Open your eyes and look at the word on the paper again. (Show the word you have written down.) Is it the same as what you saw on your mental white board? Look closely and then close your eyes again and look up and to your left and look back at the word on your mental white board, just where it was before. Great! Can you see all the letters? Are there any missing? If there are, open your eyes and have another look at the word on the page and check that you know which letters need to go in the gaps and then close your eyes again and pop them in the gaps. Excellent. Well done.

---

* Dilts, Robert & Epstein, Todd (1995) Dynamic Learning. Meta Publications.

Now tell me the very last letter you can see on your white board. Great. By the way, can you remember that nice feeling of being very pleased with yourself? Make sure you're feeling it right now. Now tell me the letter next to that one. (Continue until the client has spelled the entire word backwards. This ensures that he or she is seeing the word as an image because it would be impossible to spell backwards using a phonic method.)

Fantastic. You are brilliant. Now do it again. Start at the end and spell the word backwards. (If he or she should make a mistake, have the person re-check against the word on the page and then close his or her eyes again and put in the right letter.)

Great, you see when you spell using your eyes to see it in this way you can be a great speller! Now close your eyes, look up to your left and see the whole word again. Got it? Good, now spell it from the beginning to the end. Very well done indeed!

Tips for seeing and learning the spelling in the mind's eye

- Look upward and to the left (or to the right if the client is left handed).
- Remind the client frequently of the positive feeling of confidence and success.
- Make the letters bigger.
- If there is a letter or a cluster of letters that he or she has trouble with, get the client to make those particular letters bigger and perhaps a different colour so they really stand out from the rest.
- If it is a very long word, break it into smaller chunks that go together, e.g.

   dic **tion** ary

Learning and Exams Script: Magic bus (Be confident for class work and tests)

Age range: adaptable to age 6–9 years

Helps children let go of worries about tests (or class work) and feel more confident.

Imagine you're standing at the bus stop waiting for a bus … it's not just any old bus you know … it's a very special bus that is going to take you on a little journey to meet Spiderman/Optimus Prime/Harry Potter/any hero meaningful to the child in question … and that's not the only reason it's a special bus …

but you'll find out about that in a minute … this is a very bright, colourful bus by the way … and it's got a very smiley face on the front of it … can you see it yet? Nod your head when you can … oh great … when it draws up to the bus stop you can climb on and give your ticket to the driver … the ticket's got your name on it and it's in your pocket. … 'Oh hello (Child's Name)', says the driver … 'I've been expecting you … there's a special seat right in the front of the bus just for you … because *you are very special yourself* … hold on tightly and we'll go for a ride.'

Look out of the window … can you see that everything is changing colour … the road … is it yellow or gold? And the pavement/sidewalk is the colour of your favourite sweets/candy … I told you this is a very special bus … *just right for a very special boy/girl like you* … and can you hear there's some music playing? … I think it's your favourite song … how amazing … and just driving along … the movement of the bus seems to make you *feel very comfy and very relaxed* … yes … *you're feeling very comfy and relaxed* … and notice now that the bus is slowing down at the next bus stop … there's a big sign there … I can't quite make it out … what does it say? … Oh yes … it says '*All Worries Get Off Here*' … Is there anyone on the bus with any worries or nervous/anxious feelings? … (Child's Name) you told me you had a few worries about that test you are going to take … can you see that big dustbin by the bus stop? Just hop off for a minute and *put any old worry or nervous feeling right in the bin* where it deserves to be … just throw it in and *say goodbye to it* … and *notice how wonderful it feels without it* … brilliant … is there anything else you want to leave in there … any other bad feeling you don't want … okay put that in too and then get back on the bus … oh you look great … *you look lighter and brighter and altogether happier* … fantastic!

Okay let's sit down again … can you feel now how bouncy the seat is? … Or is it you that is so bouncy now you have thrown away those old heavy feelings into the bin? Look out of the window and when you see the Spiderman/Optimus Prime/Harry Potter/other hero stop ring the bell and get ready to jump off … nod your head when you can see it … great (Child's Name) have you rung the bell? … Look, (Hero's Name) is there to meet you and help you off the bus … the bus is going to wait for you so you can take as long as you like … shake his/her hand … and there's a little bench for you to sit on right there.

Did you know by the way that once upon a time (Hero's Name) used to be a bit nervous about tests but that he/she found a very special way to be very confident/strong/brave/relaxed/calm and he's/she's going to give you a present that will help you to feel just as confident as he/she is now … you can't actually see it but when you hold out your hands … perhaps you can feel the tingle in your fingers when you receive this amazing present … hey, can you *feel it tingling in your fingers right now*?

It's the most amazing present … it's the very special ability to *feel calm and relaxed and confident whenever you take a test* or exam or do something special at school where you really want to *feel that calm confident feeling …*

223

brilliant … isn't that wonderful … you can have this feeling whenever you want it now … whether it's for spelling or writing or reading or drawing or math(s) … you just have this amazing calm and confident feeling as soon as you open the book/look at the page/pick up your pen or pencil … and as soon as you open the book/look at the page/pick up your pen or pencil … you just *enjoy the test all the way through* … wonderful.

Listen, the driver's calling you (Child's Name). It's time to go … quickly get back on to the bus … oh look, (Hero's Name) is going with you … he's sitting down beside you … now, remember I told you this is a special bus? … It's going to drive into the future … look out of the window and tell me when you see your school … it's the day of the test … look out and see (Child's Name) going into the classroom … looking so bright and happy … see how you are so relaxed and confident … brilliant … notice how, as soon as you open the book/look at the page/pick up your pen or pencil … you just *enjoy the test all the way through* … well done (Child's Name). You are absolutely brilliant … what a good thing you left all those old feelings in the bin and (Hero's Name) gave you that wonderful present … I hope you remembered to say thank you because you can keep that for the rest of your life.

By the way, have you noticed that the bus is turning around? … I think it's time to go home … yes, we're coming back to (Hero's Name) stop … listen, he's/she's got something to say … 'Goodbye (Child's Name). It's been great to meet you … *you're a great kid* and you can just *enjoy every test you ever take from now on* … if you ever want to visit me again just close your eyes and get on the special bus (had you guessed it was a magic bus?) and go all the way home … feeling so good now … well done.

'(Child's Name) every day you will find you are more and more confident … you are very proud of the way you can do any test feeling calm and confident, and you just know deep down inside that you will do your very best.'

So I think it's time to get off the bus now and find that those sleepy dreamy feelings have been lifted right off you … and you are beginning to feel all the energy coming back into your whole body … into your toes … your feet are wanting to wriggle about … just like your hands and arms are wanting to have a big stretch and come right back to the room with me … well done (Child's Name).

Learning and Exams Script: Overcome exam nerves for older children

Age range: approximately 12 years upward. Also suitable for younger children with adaptations to specific vocabulary and ideas in order to use with younger children.

This is a prompt sheet from which you can select suggestions that are appropriate to the age and situation of the child in question rather than using the full script. You will notice that there is reference to a finger and thumb anchor. If you choose to use this, you will need to spend some time beforehand setting it up. These suggestions are appropriate for children taking relatively formal tests or exams.

You get up in the morning of your exam and you feel well rested and calm because you have slept quietly calm all night through.

You get up and you go through your normal routine with calm and ease making sure you eat breakfast to give you the energy you need for the day.

You continue feeling calm and at ease, calm in your body, calm in your mind as you gather together all the pens, pencils, etc. you need, all the things you prepared the previous day.

Whether your exams are in the morning or afternoon, you remain calm and at ease all over, all the way through the day.

Whenever you want an extra bit of calm you lightly press your finger and thumb together and feel an increased steadiness and calm come over your whole mind and body.

You go to school/college and on the journey you find your mind is drifting on to something pleasant and you remain calm and at ease.

When you arrive at the examination room, if you notice any slight extra energy, you will know this is good because you need energy to channel into developing an alert focus for your exam.

As you walk in to the room and find your place, your mind and your body are calm and at ease. You sit down and wait steadily and calmly until you are told to begin.

As you turn over the paper/open the booklet you experience a feeling of calm, alert focus.

As you pick up your pen/pencil this focus develops even more so you are completely focused as you read **each** question through thoroughly.

You see things clearly. You choose which questions are easiest for you to answer. You look for and focus on the relevant parts of the question.

Your head is clear, you think clearly and well.

You remember all of the examination skills effortlessly. Without even trying, you remember the best ways to focus your attention, read the questions carefully, make notes, write down key words related to what you want to put in your answer and stay focused on giving the answer required.

You decide how much time to spend on each question and you stick to this time, leaving yourself plenty of time for more challenging questions.

You stay calm and in control whatever the question; some questions may be more appealing than others but you stay calm and in control whether you like the question or not. You simply get on with answering the question and you are easily able to stay calm, focused and in control.

You do the very best you can with any question whether you like it or not and you usually do like it; you are calm and in control. Sometimes you seem to hear your inner voice reminding you that you are calm and in control.

You stay on track all the way through, you stick to time. You feel good, you feel calm and you channel any extra energy into alert focus that helps your concentration.

You remember to save enough time to check through your work with calm and care.

Any time you want any extra calm, you press your thumb and finger lightly together and feel that wonderful sense of calm spreading all the way through your body. Feel it now. Imagine the colour of calm spreading all the way through you, all the way through your body and mind, that wonderful colour of calm and comfort filling you up. That's right. Calm, steady, comfortable and focused. Brilliant.

So, now is the time for you to begin to reorient to the room, bringing with you the calm and composure inside. Calm and composed in your body, calm and composed in your mind. This will stay with you all through the day.

So, coming back to the room now … I am going to count from 1 to 10. Each number will bring you wider and wider awake. Each number will increase your calm and confidence … 1, you are confident … 2, you are calm and composed … 3, you are wider and wider awake … 4, you have all the energy you need … 5, you are focused and alert … 6, you are calm and you channel your energy into alert focus … 7, you feel comfortable with yourself … you are calm and composed … 8, you are calm and confident … 9, you are fully wide awake … 10, Brilliant you are wide, wide awake, fully calm and alert … thinking clearly and calmly … You feel good about yourself and the world around you.

References and Useful Resources

Chapter One: A Solution-Focused Approach

Useful books on the subject of solution-focused therapy

Furman, Ben and Ahola, Tapani. (1992) *Solution Talk: Hosting Therapeutic Conversations*. W.W. Norton.

Hawkes, David; Marsh, Trevor I; Wilgosh, Ron. (1998) *Solution Focused Therapy*. Butterworth-Heinemann.

O'Connell, Bill (1998) *Solution Focused Therapy*. Sage.

de Shazer, S. (1985) *Keys to Solution in Brief Therapy*. W.W. Norton.

de Shazer, S. (1988) *Clues Investigating Solutions in Brief Therapy*. W.W. Norton.

For those interested in solution-focused therapy, please read anything by the following authors: Steve de Shazer, Insoo Kim Berg, Ben Furman, Bill O'Hanlon, Yvonne Dolan, Michelle Weiner Davis or Mathew D. Selekman.

Origin of the miracle question

www.solutionforwardchange.blogspot.com/2007/10/who-invented-miracle-question.html
Reproduced from this site with kind permission © 1997–2008 Coert Visser – Solution-Focused Change

To my knowledge, the miracle question was first mentioned in Steve de Shazer's 1988 book *Clues: Investigating Solutions in Brief Therapy*. In this book he calls the miracle question an adaptation of Milton Erickson's crystal ball technique (in which the client is invited to create a representation of the future in which the problem was solved and then to look backwards from the future and explain how the problem had been solved).

Tapio Malinen mentions a few different accounts of how the miracle question was invented:

- An account by a certain Wilks in (Kiser, 1995, p. 136) suggests that Steve de Shazer invented it.

- According to Weiner-Davis, Eve Lipchik was the first in the work team who used this question.

- Scott Miller and Insoo Kim Berg in *Miracle Method* (1995) say the miracle question was invented when a certain client said: 'My problem is so serious that it will take a miracle to solve it!' Following her lead, the therapist simply said, 'Well, suppose one happened...?'

This last account is confirmed in 1996 by Steve de Shazer in an interview saying:

> The Miracle Question evolved out of one day Insoo asking a question and the answer was 'Oh it would take a miracle!' and Insoo said 'Well yes, suppose ... suppose a miracle did happen' ... and that started the whole thing. The answer was pretty nice, whatever it was .. the answer was nice. So. Almost all our stuff like that is invented by clients first.

Insoo once personally confirmed to me this indeed was the way the miracle question was invented. By the way, elsewhere in the same interview Steve said about Insoo's influence:

> Well, everything that we do over the years is trying to figure out how she and her clients did it. She is the Master. I don't know what other word to use. She is the Master. So all this stuff – what it really is about is attempts to describe what she and her clients do in such a way that other people – first me – the rest of the team – can do it.

All in all my interpretation is: the miracle question was invented by Insoo Kim Berg (while talking to her client), further developed by many of the members of the Brief Family Therapy Center and first published by Steve de Shazer.

Chapter Two: Inductions

'Does it *start at the top of your head and go all the way down your body*, down to the very tips of your toes? ... or, is it the other way around, do your feet get warmer first and then let the comfy feelings spread all the way up to the top of your head?' This phrase was inspired by a very similar one used by Del Hunter Morrill and used here with her permission.

Hunter Morrill, Del (2000–2004) *Great Escapes Script Series for Those Who Work with Children and Pre-Teens*, Vols. 1–4. New Beginnings.

Thanks to Juliette Howe for her suggestion of the Land of Sweets.

Chapter Three: Ego Strengthening and Self-esteem

An Overview of Self Concept Theory for Counselors, Highlights: An ERIC CAPS Digest. www.ericdigests.org

Geldard, Kathryn and Geldard, David (1997) *Counselling Children.* Sage.

Chapter Four: Nocturnal Enuresis

See the useful websites section

Chapter Five: Encopresis

'Poo in the toilet' is inspired very directly from White and Epston's (1990) idea of 'Sneaky Poo'.

Freeman, Jennifer; Epston, David; Lobovits, Dean (1997) *Playful Approaches to Serious Problems.* W.W. Norton.

White, Michael (1984) Pseudo-encopresis: from avalanche to victory, from vicious to virtuous cycles. *Family Systems Medicine*, 2:150–160). Reprinted in M. White and D. Epston (1997) *Retracing the Past: Selected Papers and Collected Papers Revisited.* Dulwich Centre Publications.

White, Michael and Epston, David (1990) *Narrative Means to Therapeutic Ends.* W.W. Norton.

They talk about the process of externalisation and how it helps to remove the idea of blame and shift the attitude of a child in therapy thus freeing them up to talk about the problem.

Chapter Six: Tics and Habits

See the useful websites section

Chapter Seven: Anxiety

James, Ursula (2005) *Clinical Hypnosis Textbook.* Radcliffe Publishing.

See the useful websites section

Chapter Eight: Separation Anxiety

See the useful websites section

Chapter Nine: Obsessive Thoughts and Compulsive Actions

Erickson, Milton H. (1998) *Life Reframing in Hypnosis*, Volume 1. Edited by Ernest L. Rossi and Margaret O' Ryan. Free Association Books.

See the useful websites section

Chapter Ten: Sleeping Difficulties

Agargu, M. et al. (2004) Sleeping position, dream emotions, and subjective sleep quality. *Sleep-and-Hypnosis.* Vol 6 (1): 8–13.

Griffin, Joe and Tyrrell, Ivan (2003) *Human Givens: A New Approach to Emotional Health and Clear Thinking.* HG Publishing.

Chapter Eleven: Being Bullied

Atkins, Sue (2007) *Raising Happy Children for Dummies.* Wiley.
Very helpful and easy to read book for parents with a section on bullying

Lovegrove, Emily (2006) *Help! I'm Being Bullied.* Accent Press.
Invaluable, practical and highly readable book with separate chapters for both children and parents.

O'Hare, Mick (2006) *Why Don't Penguins' Feet Freeze? And 114 Other Questions.* Profile Books.
Good for useful trivia.

Kidscape. www.kidscape.org.uk

McGlynn, Mary. mary@mcglynn.fsb.co.uk
Mary is a holistic therapist with a practice in Derbyshire. She uses various techniques to enable her clients to achieve integration. Her main areas of specialisation are personal development, self-esteem and relationship issues. She is also a freelance lecturer on hypnosis.

Thanks to Mary for her idea of colour breathing which I first heard about during her lecture on inner child work for the London College of Clinical Hypnosis.

Russell, Julian. PPD Consulting Ltd. www.ppdconsulting.com
Thanks to Julian for his idea of storing our best exhibits in the museum of our mind.

Chapter Twelve: Behaviour Problems

Thanks to both Ben, who was helped to manage his ADHD and Carolyn, his foster carer, for allowing me to discuss Ben's case and for permission to reproduce their comments.

See the useful websites section

Chapter Thirteen: Learning and Exams

Buzan, Tony (2003) *Mind Maps for Kids*. HarperCollins.

Dilts, Robert and Epstein, Todd (1995). *Dynamic Learning*. Meta Publications.

Ebbinghaus, H. (1885/1962). *A Contribution to Experimental Psychology*. Appendix A: Curve and Learner Retention. Dover.
The original research on memory and the discovery of the Primary/Recency Effect by Ebbinghaus was the precursor to research on memory carried out ever since.

Everatt, John and Zabell, Claire (2000) Gender differences in dyslexia, in *The Dyslexia Handbook 2000*, edited by Ian Smythe. British Dyslexia Association (pp. 83–87).

Lawlor, Michael (1988) *Inner Track Learning*. Pilgrims Publications.

Moody, Sylvia (2004) *Dyslexia: A Teenager's Guide*. Vermillion.

O'Connor, Joseph and Seymour, John (1990) *Introducing Neuro-Linguistic Programming: The New Psychology of Personal Excellence*. Mandala.
The NLP Spelling Strategy devised by Robert Dilts is clearly explained here.

Rose, Colin (1985) *Accelerated Learning*. Accelerated Learning Systems Ltd.

May-Brenneker, Eleanor, Dyslexia Consultant (AMBDA, Dyslexia Institute Guild Member, Hon. Member BBLG). 'Tudor Manor', Beckenham Place Park, Beckenham, Kent, UK, BR3 5BP
Thanks for her input on Dyslexia.

Relaxing music: See the useful websites section

Useful Books on the Subject of Working with Children

Bryant, Mike and Mabbutt, Peter (2006) *Hypnotherapy for Dummies*. John Wiley and Sons.
Has a helpful chapter for parents dealing with explanations and expectations of hypnotherapy with children.

Freeman, Jennifer; Epston, David and Lobovits, Dean (1997) *Playful Approaches to Serious Problems*. W.W. Norton.
An amazingly helpful book.

Geldard, Kathryn and Geldard, David (1997) *Counselling Children*. Sage.

Hunter Morrill, Del (2000–2004) *Great Escapes Script Series for Those Who Work with Children and Pre-Teens*, Vols. 1–4. New Beginnings. www.hypnosisonline.com

Olness, Karen and Kohen, Daniel P. (1996) *Hypnosis and Hypnotherapy with Children*. The Guilford Press.

Selekman, Matthew D. (1997) *Solution Focused Therapy with Children*. The Guilford Press.

Thomson, Linda (2005) *Harry the Hypno-potamus*, Vols. 1–2. Crown House Publishing.

Wester, William C. and Sugarman, Laurence (2007) *Therapeutic Hypnosis with Children and Adolescents*. Crown House Publishing.

For those interested in narrative and family therapy, please read anything by the following authors: Jennifer Freeman, David Epston, Michael White, Dean Lobovits. You will not be disappointed!

Useful Websites Relating to Topics in the Book

www.firstwayforward.com
A selection of CDs with ranges for children and adults written and recorded by Lynda Hudson, the author. Helpful information on bedwetting and other childhood problems. Also details of Lynda's private practice in Beckenham, South East London.

www.enhancingvitality.com
Anne Lesley Marshall offers resource ebooks and EFT as a tool for building up confidence for kids.

Nocturnal enuresis

www.firstwayforward.com/bedwetting.html
www.eric.org.uk
www.netdoctor.co.uk

Encopresis

www.kidshealth.org
www.medicinenet.com

Tics/Tourette Syndrome

www.tourettes-action.org.uk
www.psychnet-uk.com/dsm_iv/transient_tic_disorder.htm

Anxiety and separation anxiety

www.psychiatrycpd.org/learningmodules/podcasts/
    anxietydisordersinchildren.aspx
www.ncpamd.com/anxiety.htm

Obsessions and compulsions

www.psychiatrycpd.org/learningmodules/podcasts/
    anxietydisordersinchildren.aspx
www.rcpsych.ac.uk

Bullying

www.kidscape.org.uk
A great website for parents and children. Gives excellent advice on dealing with bullying.

ADHD and ODD

www.familydoctor.org
www.Mayoclinic.com
www.netdoctor.co.uk
www.rcpsych.ac.uk

Dyslexia

www.bdadyslexia.org.uk
www.dyslexia.uk.com
Dyslexia Research Trust: www.dyslexic.org.uk

Accelerated learning

www.acceleratedlearning.co.uk

www.anglo-american.co.uk: an excellent selection of recent publications on thinking, learning, mind mapping and teaching using accelerated learning principles.

Music suitable for relaxing and as background to studying

www.tonyoconnor.com.au
www.innerpeacemusic.com

Parents and children

www.kidscape.org.uk
Great informative website for parents and children.

Training Organisations

www.lcch.co.uk

The London College of Clinical Hypnosis, Clinical Hypnotherapy Training, founded by Michael Joseph. Courses available in UK, Europe and Asia, accredited by Thames Valley University

www.thamesmedicallectures.com

Thames Medical Lectures, led by Ursula James FBAMH, is a unique organisation delivering high quality, individually tailored training courses to the medical profession.

www.isiscentre.co.uk

A training course in hypnosis, psychotherapy and Neuro Linguistic Programming (NLP) led by Christina Mills, founder and director, and Christopher Fish, director.

www.cityminds.com

Innovative workshops and programmes for parents, students, schools and teachers. Maggie Chapman and Avy Joseph are directors and co founders.

www.itsnlp.com

International Teaching Seminars (ITS) was established in 1988 by Ian McDermott and provides high quality NLP training. The focus is on practical applications of NLP and the importance of personal congruence in implementing it.

www.gil-boyne.com

Gil Boyne, often linked with Erickson and Elman as one of the pioneers of modern hypnotherapy, gives masterclasses in Advanced Training in Clinical Hypnotherapy. He is now based in London, UK.

www.hypnosiseire.com

Training in Ireland: Institute of Clinical Hypnotherapy & Psychotherapy, led by Dr Joe Keaney.

Hypnotherapy Associations

www.bsch.org.uk

The British Society of Clinical Hypnosis (BSCH) is a national professional body whose aim is to promote and assure high standards in the practice of hypnotherapy. You can search for a therapist with good quality training, ethical practice and adherence to the code of conduct.

www.general-hypnotherapy-register.com

The General Hypnotherapy Register (GHR) of Hypnotherapists in the UK is open to those who satisfy GHR training and on-going requirements. It promotes unity, maintenance of good practice and continuing professional development within the profession of hypnotherapy.

Index

Accelerated learning   206–209, 231,
   234
   Active reading   209
   Associations   207
   Colour   207, 220
   Linked stories   208
   Primary/Recency Effect   209, 231
   Mind Maps   208, 231
   Mnemonics   208
   Music   208
   Problems   211
   Tactile/kinaesthetic
      strategies   207, 221
   Working in short bursts   209
Achievement scenario   5, 7–8, 10
Agargu, M.   165, 230
Anchors   38, 100, 110, 131, 176
Antidiuretic Hormone (ADH)   45
Anxiety   46, 95–123
   Association and generalisation   97
   Avoidance   97
   Component parts   95
   Nature of   95, 98
   Origins   47, 96–97
   Reinforcement   97
Attention Deficit Hyperactivity
      Disorder (ADHD)   78–80, 191,
      192, 196, 197, 205, 210, 231, 233

Bedwetting   6, 29, 45, 232, 233;
      see also Enuresis
Behaviour problems   31, 191–204,
      231
Berg, Insoo Kim   5, 227, 228
Blasphemous or obscene
      thoughts   138
Body Focused Repetitive Behaviours
      (BFRBs)   151
Breathing:
   Controlled   101
   Cupped hands   102
   Ratio   102

Brief Family Therapy Center   5, 228
Bullying   29–32, 47, 63, 80, 128, 164,
      173–189
   Effects of   173–174
   Physical danger   176
   Types of   173–174, 187
   Victim thinking   175, 177

Common childhood
      apprehensions   99
Coping strategies   63, 153
   Calm triggers   104
   Challenging the thoughts   104
   Coping statements   104
Colon clearing   66
Conduct disorder   62
Confusional reframe   170
Constipation   48, 59
   Causes   62–63
   Consequences   63–64
   Physical and emotional
      aspects   63
   Signs   60
   Withholding   63, 65
Contamination (fear of)   138
Coprololalia   79
Copropraxia   79

Deep sleep   47
Deliberate soiling   62, 66
Depotentiating the thought   141
Desmopressin (DDAVP)   48
Dissociation   37, 105, 106, 108, 109,
      154, 164
Disturbing dreams   99, 126, 163–166
Dyscalculia   210
Dyslexia   205, 210–213, 231, 233
Dyspraxia   210

EARS procedure   12
Echolalia   79
Echopraxia   79

Ego strengthening   29–43, 52, 64, 66, 122, 140, 165, 176, 198, 206
   Compliments   10, 30, 41
   Confidence   32, 33, 49, 51, 80, 100, 108, 110, 126, 153, 175, 205, 213, 222–232
Emotional stress   46, 63
Encopresis   59–76, 229, 233
Enuresis, nocturnal   45–58, 229, 233
   Causes   45–47
   Conventional treatment   48–49
   Physical problems   46
   Slow development of regulatory systems   46
   Small functional bladder capacity   46
Epston, David   67, 229, 232
Erickson, Milton   141, 230, 235
Euphemisms   158
Everatt, John   211, 231
Exam nerves   205–226
Externalisation   67, 76, 159, 229

Faecal impaction   60
Faecal incontinence   60
Fear:
   of the dark   161, 170
   of monsters   63, 160, 162–163
Freeman, Jennifer   67, 229, 232

Geldard, David   30, 229, 232
Geldard, Kathryn   30, 229, 232
Generalised Anxiety Disorder (GAD)   98
Genetics   96, 137
Griffin, Joe   163, 230
Group A Beta-Hemolytic Streptococcal (GABHS) infection   80

Habits; *see* Tics
Homework activities   10–12
Hopwood, Larry   5
Hypno-desensitisation   121–122

Imipramine Hydrochloride   48
Inductions   15–27, 100, 176–178, 196–198, 228
Irritable Bowel Syndrome (IBS)   65

James, Ursula   121, 229, 234

Kidscape   174, 230, 233, 234

Learning and exams   205–226, 231
Legal and safety procedures   4
Lobovits, Dean   67, 229, 232

Miller, Scott   5, 228
Miracle question   227, 228

Neuro Linguistic Programming (NLP)   2, 10, 38, 140–142, 213, 221, 231, 234
Nightmares   99, 126, 163–166
NLP Spelling Strategy   221, 231

Obsessive Compulsive Disorder (OCD)   78–80, 98, 100, 137, 138, 140, 153
Obsessive Compulsive Personality Disorder (OCPD)   138
Obsessive thoughts and compulsive actions   137–155, 230
   Common obsessive thoughts, urges, images, fears and anxieties   138–139
   Compulsive actions and rituals   139
Oppositional Defiant Disorder (ODD)   62, 191, 192

Paediatric Autoimmune Neuropsychiatric Disorders Associated with Streptococcal Infections (PANDAS)   79
Panic disorder   99
Post-Traumatic Stress Disorder (PTSD)   98–99, 127
Protective pants   47, 49

Rewind procedure   100, 105–108, 164, 165, 264
Right-side sleepers   165
Ritalin   197
Rituals   137, 139–140, 197

Scaling   195
Self-concept   29–32, 33, 229
Self-esteem   29–32, 51, 62, 64, 66, 80, 100, 126, 127, 153, 174, 175, 177, 195, 205, 229
Separation Anxiety   98, 125–135
  Handout   129
  Onset   125
  Signs   126
  Symptoms   127–128
  Tips for parents and caregivers   129
Shazer, Steve de   5, 227, 228
Sleeping difficulties   157–171
  Night sounds   160
  Worrying thoughts and feelings   157–159
Sleeping positions   165, 230
Social phobia   98
Soiling   6, 29, 59, 61–62, 229
Solution-Focused Approach   1–13, 193, 227
Strep throat   80, 138
Study handout   220
Subjective Units of Disturbance Scale (SUDS)   122
Suggestion, direct and indirect   140–141
Supportive messages   12

Temper   192–194
Tests and exams   206, 222, 224
Tics   77–94
  Characteristics   77–78
  Chronic   78
  Medication   79
  Motor   77
  Premonitory urges   89
  Spectrum   79
  Transient   78
  Vocal   77
Toilet training   62, 66, 68
Tourette Syndrome (TS)   78, 233
Tourette, Dr Georges Gilles de la   78
Trichophagia   152
Trichobezoars   152
Trichotillomania (TTM)   138, 151, 153, 154
Tyrrell, Ivan   163, 230

Unwanted thoughts   127, 137, 140–142, 159

Vasopressin   46
Visual hierarchy of fears   123

Writing induction scripts for young people:
  Age groups   17–18
  Embedded suggestions   15
  Engagement   16
  Gender   17
  Metaphorical stories   15

Zabell, Claire   211, 231

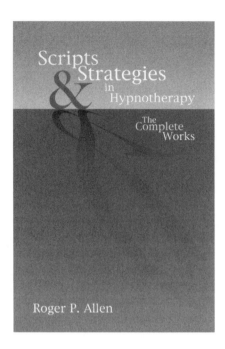

Scripts and Strategies in Hypnotherapy

The Complete Works

Roger P Allen

ISBN: 978-190442421-5

Roger P. Allen's *Scripts and Strategies in Hypnotherapy: The Complete Works* presents a comprehensive source of scripts and strategies that can be used by hypnotherapists to build a successful framework for any therapy session.

This book – or, to be more specific, this revised and updated compendium of Volumes I and II – is designed to be of assistance to all therapists as they unlock the possibilities that exist for their clients and help them make significant and beneficial changes to their perceptions and beliefs. Upon compiling it, Allen's ultimate aim was to provide practitioners with the best toolkit of strategies possible, replete with a variety of practical scripts to serve as the basis for their interventions, derived from his own experiences as a therapist.

It covers inductions, deepeners and actual scripts for a wide range of cases; from nail biting to insomnia, sports performance to past life recall, speech difficulty to loss and bereavement, pain management to resolving sexual problems, and more. There is a particularly comprehensive section on smoking cessation, including a specimen questionnaire for use during the initial interview as well as useful content for a leaflet on the dangers of smoking to give to clients to take away with them following the session.

All of the scripts can be used as they stand, or adapted as necessary for specific situations and for client-specific needs and concerns.

Suitable for hypnotherapists of all levels of experience.